FOUR MINUTES
to LIFE

Other Books by ANN CUTLER

TRACHTENBERG SPEED SYSTEM OF
BASIC MATHEMATICS

INSTANT MATH

FOUR MINUTES to LIFE

by ANN CUTLER

COWLES BOOK COMPANY, INC.
NEW YORK

Photos pp. 154-156, 158-162,
© New York State Department of Health, 1966

Photos pp. 165-167,
Courtesy American Heart Association

Photos pp. 168-169,
Courtesy Smith Kline & French Laboratories

CONTENTS

FOREWORD

by
JAMES R. JUDE, M.D.
Chief of Cardiovascular Surgery, University of Miami
Medical School

The foreboding barrier into death that all must cross is today only a premature visit for some people. Such transitory passage has become commonplace in today's world of miracle medicine. Suspended animation, a description in neoscientific medicine of quasi-death, is a common and reversible state today. This is the time between clinical death (loss of external pulse and breathing) and biological death (where cellular biochemical changes are irreversible). The miracle of resuscitation is not so much that biological death can be thwarted, but by whom this can be done. The simplification of sustaining and reinstitution of both heartbeat and respiration has given to paramedical personnel and even the layman this awesome power.

The potential for saving lives with resuscitation is enormous. The majority of reversible sudden deaths occur outside the hospital. A high percentage of these victims of sudden death could be saved if laymen—who are usually the first on the scene of an accident, electrocution, drowning, asphyxia, or death from a sudden heart attack—were able to give immediate resuscitation.

For the victim of sudden death, there is only four minutes before irreversible death (biological cellular death) sets in. This critical period of time makes all important the need for immediate action. To drastically cut the appalling number of premature deaths, resuscitation of the heart and lungs needs the combined efforts of the medical profession plus the dedicated cooperation of the public.

From the description of breathing life into the dead boy as described in the Second Book of Kings, through to the evolvement of modern medical scientific thought of the late nineteenth century, the ability of physicians to restore life has emerged. Mouth-to-mouth respiration became scientifically accepted in the early 1950s, but it was in the exciting laboratory of Dr. William Kouwenhoven that in late 1957 there fell the real emergence of nonoperative resuscitation of the heart.

There it was discovered by doctoral student G. Guy Knickerbocker that the rhythmic pressure by the hand on the breastplate could keep the heart of an animal alive even though the heart had ceased to beat. One year later, a woman was brought in one late evening to the operating room of the Johns Hopkins Hospital for emergency gall bladder surgery. During the early phases of anesthesia, her heart action stopped and the external heart compression technique was applied for the first time to a human being. The restoration of spontaneous and effective heart contraction proved the method to be an astonishing success.

By mid-1960, a great many effective results could be reported to the medical world. And so, there came about a simple heart resuscitation method with applicability not then truly realized.

Ann Cutler has brought together, brilliantly and dramatically, the developments that have changed the phenomenon of death and even its definition; the reversible problems of asphyxia and cardiac arrest; the problems of delayed resuscitation and brain damage; the ability of man to sustain a biological "life" without brain function, as well as the expense and fruitlessness of prolongation of such existence. Miss Cutler's background in the study of such medical miracles as that of the recovery of Landau has given her unusual insight into the relationship of such accomplishments to the commonplace existence of reversible death.

Diseases of the heart and blood vessels account for the final exodus of more Americans than all other diseases combined. Coronary artery disease alone has reached epidemic proportions as it takes upwards of 700,000 lives annually in the United States. And tragically the death grip of coronary occlusion edges toward younger and younger age groups. More than 50 percent of sudden deaths from this cause occur outside the hospital before the physician's aid can be obtained.

Utilizing the techniques of resuscitation, sudden heart stoppage is being treated successfully outside of the hospital by specialized ambulances staffed by highly trained lay rescue squads. Radio telemetry conveys electrocardiograms and physicians' instructions are relayed in return. The in-hospital coronary care units have dropped the death rate for those fortunate enough to reach them.

It is the early, the untoward death, the faltering of the flower of life that medical science is striving to eliminate. Ann Cutler has captured the exciting aura of man's assist to God's hand in preserving the flicker of the heartbeat's warmth of life. Captured, too, are the hopelessness, the frustrations of these efforts, for ultimately—as with her account of Dr. Landau—it is only a temporary restraining of the ultimate accomplishment of life's eternal cycle.

1.
WHAT IS DEATH?

All through the expanse of time death has been unchallenged. Until this century modern science did little probing into the phenomenon of death. Surrounded by superstition and fear, it was a taboo subject. Yet death is a significant clinical event. The first constructive research on the subject was begun by scientists during World War II. They found that death, like any disease, had physical and biochemical components. Studying how people die, scientists have learned a great deal about how to make people live.

Until recently man has always felt his destiny was foreordained the minute he was conceived. In many ways he was right, for at that moment he received much of the physical, mental, and emotional equipment he was to carry through life. And he could almost forecast his life span by the existence period enjoyed by his ancestors. If he came from healthy, long-living stock, he had a good chance of surviving longer than those whose origin was rooted in backgrounds where disease, illness, and weakness consistently shortened the life span.

The specter of death shaped much of man's philosophy, played a vital role in religion, and to a great extent dictated man's economy. The inevitability of death was at the root of his despair as well as the basis for his sense of irony. Living with the knowledge that his existence on earth amounted to only a brief interval, man made his plans accordingly.

But eternal youth and life everlasting has always been one of the dreams of mankind—the promise made by all religions. The ancients lusted for the elixir of youth. Conquistadores braved mountains and deserts in search of the promised fountains. Wistfully they decided they were a mirage, a wish of the human heart that could not be fulfilled.

Today some of the finest medical minds in the world are working toward the day when death can be held off indefinitely. As recently as a decade ago, there was no turning back when death struck. Now thousands of men, women, and children have been restored to life, their deaths reversed by the new methods of resuscitation.

It is now common among medical practitioners to make a distinction between *clinical death* and *biological death*. Clinical death is that state which sets in immediately after the heart stops and respiration ceases. Biological death—when the whole organism has deteriorated to such a degree that there is no possibility of salvage—follows within minutes unless swift steps are taken to reverse the outcome.

Clinical death, which resembles total death and which the law recognizes as such, is actually a transitional state between life and death. There are at this time still elements of life which, though difficult to discern, yet may serve as the basis of resuscitation. For the body does not die all at once. There is an order and system in death as there is in all phases of life.

The first organ to die biologically is the brain, followed by the respiratory organs. The spinal cord comes next. The heart is the last bulwark of life—the last to die. When resuscitation takes place, the heart is the first to come back.

The discovery that the transition from life to death is a lengthy process and not a momentary leap made obsolete the ancient conception of death. The new, successful methods of resuscitation that range all the way from mouth-to-mouth breathing and closed-heart massage to the transplant of hearts and the use of hypothermia—the technique of artificial cooling— have made "the distinction between life and death grow increasingly less distinct," says Dr. John S. Flick, Jr., a Philadelphia surgeon.

What is death?

Death has always appeared to be a relatively simple and clearly definable end to life. It came when a man stopped breathing and his heart ceased beating. Today this definition is inaccurate, for there is no longer anything absolute about death. When a man stops breathing and his heart stops beating, he is not yet dead but only unable to *personally* sustain life.

The question "Is he dead?" has been replaced by "Can he be brought back to life?" In many cases artificial respiration and cardiac massage can restore him to life. That death is reversible is demonstrated countless times every day by first-aid squads and lifeguards as well as doctors.

More and more doctors now argue that life terminates when the brain permanently ceases to function—even though the heartbeat and respiration may be sustained by artificial respirators. They urge that death be ascertainable by electroencephalogram (EEG or "brain waves") readings. For today it is widely acknowledged that the human spirit is the product of man's brain, not of his heart.

But even this definition may prove temporary. French Academy member Jean Rostand states that as a criterion of death, prolonged interruption of the electrical activity of the brain may become outmoded in the future.

"A dead man is only temporarily incurable," says Dr. Rostand. "The notion of physiological death has changed through the years and it is possible that a man considered dead in 1969 might not be considered dead if he were in the year 2000."

Today scientists are already working toward the time when death can be delayed indefinitely. Experts in gerontology—the science of the biology of aging—say it is definitely within the realm of possibility that before the end of this century death will have been conquered—or at least held at bay for longer and longer periods.

Dr. Bernard Strehler, of the National Institute of Health at

Bethesda, Maryland, an expert in the field of g ontology, recently stated:

> There is little doubt among those who are most active in re-
> search in the field that an understanding of the biology of aging
> is within the reach of this generation provided that a sufficient
> priority in terms of good brains, sound financing, adequate
> facilities, and administrative support is given this undertaking.

Scientists have long believed that man's life expectancy
should be eight times his age at maturity—as is the case of all animals. A dog is fully grown at two years of age and has a life expectancy of sixteen years; a horse matures at four and lives until
he is thirty-two. Man, who becomes physically mature at the age
of twenty-five, should, therefore, have a life expectancy of two
hundred years.

But now that it looks as if the promise of unlimited survival is
about to be redeemed, there is uneasiness and fear. The idea of
tampering with the life cycle awakens old forebodings. However, it is axiomatic that in medicine the miracles of yesterday
are the common practices of today and the mysteries of today
may be the common knowledge of tomorrow.

Psychiatrists point out that the desire to avoid death is normal
and that the seizing of even a slim chance to survive in prefer-
ence to none is rational.

If medical science makes it possible for man to live for centuries, the terms of his thinking and planning will have to be
drastically changed, for it will affect greatly the socio-economic
structure of our society. The repercussions of altering a man's
life will be moral, legal, and ethical.

The use of resuscitative techniques in the fight against death,
say its defenders, is not in any way contradictory to the teach-
ings of religion, for it does not renew life but extends it, much
as our new miracle drugs and brilliant surgical innovations do.

Nor will prolonging the life cycle have a disastrous effect on
our already exploding population. It has been pointed out that
the population problem cannot be solved by killing people,

either by commission or omission. To refuse a person medical care, including resuscitation at death, would be tantamount to sentencing him to death without reprieve. The solution to the population problem lies in birth control and in an expanding economy.

The reason for the fearful approach to lengthening man's life span is that the public in general does not understand science and is not aware either of its capabilities or how its wondrous accomplishments are achieved. Thus they remain ignorant of the forces that are shaping their future.

New and surprising discoveries are often met with shock or at least dubious approval. Even the simpler devices that civilization has produced were effective only when the science behind them was fully understood.

Dr. Lev Davidovich Landau, famous Nobel Prize-winning scientist of the Soviet, addressing the International Congress of High Energy Particles in 1959, might have been talking of the new scientific attitude toward death when he said: "Conservatism must be feared more than revolutionism. The rejection of earlier ideas will, of course, be accompanied by the appearance of new ones, truer ones, and therefore more fruitful ones."

Dr. Landau went on to point out that Einstein's theory of relativity had at first seemed insane because it forced physicists to deny there was an absolute time. He then reminded the Congress that many of the startlingly new theories produced by scientists were so shattering to old beliefs that they often caused psychological traumas when first presented. Nevertheless, if the theories were good, they were finally accepted.

The twentieth century has had more scientific accomplishments than all the thousands of years that preceded it and 90 percent of all the scientists that have ever lived are still alive. That the latter part of this century will far outdistance the past is an accepted fact, for the number of scientific achievements is doubling every ten years.

Daring and bold as the explorers of another era, imaginative yet precise in their calculations, scientists are touching every aspect of life from politics to longevity, causing revolutionary changes and introducing technological discoveries that will affect mankind for all time to come. Nowhere is the public more intimately concerned than in the rapid development of medical science. Massive steps taken in this field during the past fifty years can best be emphasized by a look backward. In 1910 there were still no X rays, no cardiograms, no knowledge of basal metabolism, no antibiotics, and also no vaccines. It was almost twenty-five years before doctors began talking about viruses and learned to identify them under a microscope.

In 1910 tuberculosis was rampant under the name of consumption, coronary occlusion passed for acute indigestion, and the chief weapon against pneumonia was digitalis. In the operating theater, surgery consisted mostly of the removal of tonsils; appendectomies were scheduled for practically any pain in the abdomen. The death rate was high. Most of it was put to "God's will" since there seemed no one else to blame.

In a century where two major wars sparked a crucial need and deep interest in scientific developments of all kinds, medicine, which throughout the ages had been practiced chiefly as an art, took on new importance and brand-new character. As research accelerates at an ever-increasing rate, many of the forecasts that sound a little like fortune-telling become accomplished fact. When medical science predicts that within this decade we will have the cure for leukemia and other forms of cancer, its prognostications are not based on wishful thinking, but on knowledge of work in progress. At the National Institute of Health, where testing of drugs is routine, 284 cancer drugs were used on human beings in the last ten years. Prior to that, there were only three such drugs. And new ones are constantly being developed. The law of averages alone makes it probable that cures will be found.

Pathologists and scientists emphatically declare that no one has ever died of old age. People die of disease and accidents. This is significant, for medicine has never admitted there is a disease that is ultimately incurable. And as cures for more diseases are found, our life span will be extended far beyond the limits we know today.

"Some day we may be able to find what ages the cell and what prevents healthy cellular replacement," says Professor Frederick A. Whitehouse, of the Rehabilitation Counseling Program at Hofstra University. "For I do not believe that death is as natural as life, although to date the evidence is indeed almost infinitely strong that it is."

Molecular biology is the science that is making possible experiments with the basic chemistry of life. Scientists predict that the greatest change we are going to see in the future will be effected by the explosion of biological knowledge already taking place. They believe that by 1980 it should be possible to control diseases caused by the body's own malfunctioning, such as cancer and the allergies; that we can expect sex predetermination by 1980; and control of the aging process, enabling us to be as productive at sixty-five to seventy-five as we now are at forty-five to fifty-five. Beyond getting rid of diseases and defects, there is the prospect that science can actually improve human beings—making them more intelligent, more talented, and more virtuous—by manipulation.

"The recent progress in knowledge of gerontology, the effects of hormones, the techniques of tissue culture, the relationship between diet and atherosclerosis, and the effects of underfeeding and freezing on individual cells, keeps a distant light aflame in the ever continuing search for human longevity," says Dr. Gerald J. Gruman, assistant professor of history at the University of Massachusetts.

Many gerontologists are convinced that medicine has already provided an outline for an average life span of well over a hundred years. Recent findings seem to indicate that life can retain its vim even into the very advanced years. Just as there is no death from aging, neither is there any sudden decrepitude due solely to the aging process. Much of the deterioration once blamed on age is really due to disease. Arteriosclerosis, or hardening of the arteries, for instance, was long considered a normal aging process. But we now know it is caused by an imbalance of the body's chemistry.

The bone disease known as osteoporosis, which made people in their seventies and eighties as fragile as glass, has been all but eliminated by hormone replacement. The remarkable physical and mental effects of estrogens have already been demonstrated in middle-aged women. There is now the promise of similar hormonal age-retardants for the male.

The crucial power of the older years is the intelligence. The emphasis is on keeping the mind young along with the body. Present studies point up the fact that at an age when other generations took to the rocking chair, men and women today are finding new uses for their intelligence, imagination, and knowledge. In their fifties and sixties, with half of their adult life ahead of them, they are not ready for the shelf.

It is now known that the line of the mind does not follow the line of the body's fast growth and long, gradual decline. Instead it rises slowly, lifted by learning to a plateau that stretches across the adult years. There is a small decline with age in low IQ echelons; it is even smaller in the middle range; and in people of superior intelligence there is almost no perceptible decline. While the expression of intelligence changes, the capacity of intelligence remains.

Dr. Edward Bortz, a past president of the American Medical Association, says that the emphasis is on "living" as contrasted with existing. It is this facet of aging—adding not just years but meaningful time to the life span—that is of the greatest interest to medicine. If the spirit is willing to continue with a rich life into "old age," the flesh, fortified by modern medical understanding, is certainly strong enough to carry on, according to Dr. Bortz.

The ability to live for centuries is taken for granted in the Soviet Union, which has long conducted intensive research on longevity. Man of the future will live to be three hundred years old and will need only one hour's sleep a night, according to Soviet scientist Vladimir Engelhardt. "As soon as we know what makes man tired we will be able to slow down the process." At seventy-two years of age, Dr. Engelhardt is sure that he will live to see this and many other changes in man's way of life. He says: "By the time I am one hundred and fifty, I will have lived only half my life."

Hubert Humphrey visited the Soviet Union when he was Vice-President and became familiar with the amazing results of their work in reversing death. He later told a United States Senate committee: "No man can now foresee what a greatly enlarged scientific drive could achieve if we were to launch it. But a decade from now, we may look back to present-day attitudes toward death as 'primitive' and 'medieval' in the same way we now look upon a once-dreaded killer like tuberculosis."

Past experience has shown that those who go in for prognostication are apt to err in the direction of underestimating the capabilities of science. In 1937, for instance, several scientists were queried about what they thought life would be like in twenty-five years. The major predictions had to do with developments expected through the use of fractional horsepower—small electrical motors. They completely missed radar, space travel, antibiotics, and jet transportation—all commonplace today.

Dr. B. G. Ballard, president of the National Research Commission, makes the point that "the great breakthroughs which made our present civilization possible were not the result of solving problems that we knew about, but rather of learning the secrets of nature which made possible the solutions."

Just as the twentieth century marks a momentous breakthrough in man's exploration of outer space, so the last part of the century will open doors to extensive exploration of death and external life.

2.

SUDDEN DEATH STRIKES EVERYWHERE

At four o'clock on a bright October afternoon, a prominent attorney left his Baltimore office to attend a business conference.

He had walked only a short distance through the city's crowded business district when suddenly he was gripped by excruciating pain. The seizure caught his body in agony so intense that he could not breathe. His heart fluttered wildly, and he pitched forward heavily onto the hard pavement.

A crowd gathered. A man who was nearby pressed forward and identified himself as a doctor. The crowd parted for him. Bending over the body, he picked up the flaccid wrist of the man on the sidewalk. There was no pulse. Nor could he discern any signs of respiration.

"This man is dead!" the doctor told the onlookers. Shocked by the swiftness of tragedy, they stood motionless. Death had descended among them like a ravaging hawk, reminding them of their own vulnerability, for death is never very far away.

Suddenly an ambulance pulled up at the curb. Two firemen jumped out and ran over to the body. Someone who had seen the lawyer's death agony had put a call through for the rescue squad.

Quickly the firemen turned the man over. They could find no pulse, no respiration, no heartbeat, no reaction of the dilated pupils. All the criteria of death were present. But these men were trained in the new techniques of resuscitation.

The doctor told the rescuers the man was dead. But the young firemen did not seem to hear. The man had been dead less than three minutes. There was still a chance.

"It's our job to resuscitate," one of the firemen told the doctor. He quickly took a position near the head of the stricken man, placed his hand under the man's neck, thus throwing the head backward and creating an open airway. He covered his fingers with a clean handkerchief and deftly explored the inside of the mouth to make sure there was no obstruction. Then he took a deep breath, bent over, and placed his mouth tightly against that of the man on the sidewalk and exhaled thoroughly.

As the fireman lifted his head, he looked at the man's chest. He saw it rise and fall, the chest movement showing that oxygen was getting through to the lungs. He took another deep breath and continued his exhalations at the rate of fifteen times a minute.

The other fireman, who knelt beside the man's chest, placed the heels of his hands, one over the other, on the lower part of the breastbone. Pressing down, he manipulated the heart, pushing hard on the breastbone to start the circulation. Each manipulation compressed the chest a good two inches. Raising his hands briefly between each compression, he fell into a pattern, compressing the chest at a steady rate of sixty times a minute.

Racing the clock to save a life, the work of the two men was rhythmical and sure.

The victim soon began to breathe on his own, an initial infinitesimal breath that, after the long period of unconsciousness, seemed miraculous. It was a promise that the next breath would come and the next until the breath of life was restored. Very faintly the heart began to beat.

The crowd stood awestruck. They had witnessed a sudden and terrible death. And now they were watching a miracle—a modern resurrection. But the rescue work had just begun. It was merely the first step in a long procession of resuscitative techniques.

The man who had been doing mouth-to-mouth breathing pulled a wheeled stretcher from the ambulance. The two firemen maneuvered the still unconscious victim onto the stretcher and pushed it toward the ambulance while they continued to blow air into his lungs and manipulate his chest.

The ambulances used in Baltimore are of a new design, with high ceiling and wide body, allowing plenty of room to work. A seat, with seatbelts, is placed alongside the litter so that an attendant can always be at the side of the patient. A sophisticated array of equipment made it possible for one of the men to take the wheel while the other took over the job of resuscitation, which must be kept up during the ride to the hospital.

Placing an oxygen mask on the face of the patient, the fireman continued to compress the chest still at the rate of sixty times a minute, forcing the continuing circulation of blood through the vital areas. As he worked, he kept careful watch over the oxygen mask, seeing to it that no leakage developed. The rescuer was making sure that the victim was kept in the gray area of clinical death from which doctors would be able to bring him back to life. If he was allowed to slip into biological death, it would be forever too late.

The medical team that staffed the emergency room of the hospital had been notified by the ambulance's two-way radio that a heart patient was on the way. The fifteen members of the team were ready to go to work the instant the ambulance arrived. The patient was placed on the floor—for a hard surface is mandatory—and a cardiologist took over the arduous task of squeezing the chest. An anesthetist, whose job in resuscitation is vital, quickly inserted a plastic tube into the patient's throat, and attached it to a rubber bag which sent oxygen directly to the lungs.

Working urgently—for every second counts—the team resembled the cast of a well-rehearsed play, each knowing what must be done and doing it expertly. A doctor connected the electrocardiograph, another readied the defibrillator (a machine that sends a shock of powerful voltage through a heart that has lost its rhythm). Nurses came hurrying with trays, intravenous feeding stands, bottles of drugs.

An intern exposed a vein in the ankle and started an intravenous infusion of bicarbonate of soda to buffer the acid condition that often accompanies sudden death. Another doctor gave the patient a shot of epinephrine, a powerful drug used routinely to stimulate the heart. Throughout this procedure the heart continued to be squeezed in order to maintain circulation.

The doctor monitoring the electrocardiogram announced that the heart was fibrillating furiously (a spasm or convulsion when the heart races and jiggles but does not accomplish anything; unless fibrillation is controlled it invariably proves fatal).

"All right," the doctor performing the massage said. "Get ready!"

Two insulated electrodes, shaped like paddles, were held out by an intern. The cardiologist seized them between compressions. Positioning them on the patient's chest, he yelled "Shock!" as the current was turned on for one-tenth of a second, sending 550 volts of electricity through the fibrillating heart. Without losing his rhythm, the doctor resumed the heart massage.

Again the electrocardiogram showed erratic, wavering lines that meant fibrillation. The shock was repeated. This time it worked. The heart stopped momentarily. And then as the doctor compressed the chest, the lawyer's heart started beating on its own.

The patient opened his eyes. His pupils shifted uneasily. He did not appear to know where he was. But after a minute or two, his vague stare focused and he seemed to regain control of his consciousness. His heart beat on, more and more strongly. His breathing deepened and steadied.

But the fight was not yet finished. Death, the doctors know, grimly waits for a second chance. Only minute-by-minute care for the next five days would give the lawyer a chance to take his place among the living—for these are crucial days when many patients are lost. He was placed on a bed and moved to the Coronary Care Unit where he was hooked up to electric cardiac monitoring equipment which sends a continuous report to a central nursing station and provides instant response to an emergency. Here a second heart attack would be checked before it had time to let death win.

After the acute danger point was over, the lawyer, whom we will call John Russell, was moved to a private room. He was made, as is now thought important, to resume normal activity as soon as possible. He was allowed to sit up after the first week and before he left the hospital he was walking up and down the corridors.

Five weeks after he was carried into the emergency room, Mr. Russell left the hospital. His heart was mending. Today he is back in practice, in better health than he has been for years.

Mr. Russell was fortunate to have his heart attack in Baltimore, one of the few cities in the United States equipped to fight death at all times. In most cities he would have been carted off to a morgue, for there would have been few people with the precise knowledge of modern resuscitation to bring him back to life during the crucial moments when he was still in clinical death.

The first instruction on closed-chest resuscitation was given to a class of Baltimore firemen on May 15, 1960. Hubert A. Cheek and Marvin T. Burkindine, crewmen on ambulance number 2, participated in the class. Four days later, these two answered a call. They found a sixty-year-old man—Bert Bish —lying on a couch apparently dead. There was no discernible pulse or respiration and the man was blue.

Cheek immediately placed his hands over the victim's breast-bone and started to pump—just as he had seen the Johns Hopkins instructors demonstrate a few days before. Later Cheek told Dr. W. B. Kouwenhoven, who helped develop closed-chest massage: "I pressed on the man's chest for a few minutes and damned if he didn't breathe!"

As the ambulance sped Bish to the hospital, Cheek continued to give resuscitation. At Johns Hopkins doctors employed for the first time a new type of defibrillator—a machine that could shock the heart out of sporadic beating through a closed chest. With this type of defibrillator the patient whose heart is fibrillating does not have to withstand the trauma of having his chest cut open. The machine is now used in most hospitals throughout the country.

Eight weeks later Bish left the hospital well on the mend. Unlike most heart attack victims of that time, he had undergone no surgery and had no side effects to overcome.

Since the Bish case, all police and firemen in the city of Baltimore receive training in life-saving techniques. So do doctors, nurses, public health personnel, lifeguards, and ambulance attendants. This is why Baltimore ranks first among cities equipped to give immediate help to victims of sudden death.

The young firemen who came to Mr. Russell's rescue had undergone rigorous training in first aid to prepare for the job of *first class firefighters* (the highest rank). They had attended an ambulance school which is run under the supervision of the Johns Hopkins Institute. At the end of their training they had to pass a competitive examination in which performance tests were given by the Civil Service Commission. Among the things they had to master in order to qualify was mouth-to-mouth breathing and heart massage.

And just to make sure that the rescue workers do not get sloppy on their job, they are given a yearly retraining program. So excellent is the work of the Baltimore firemen who become rescue fighters that a doctor told a group of physicians: "If anything happens to me, I'd rather have one of the fire rescuers come to my aid than one of you."

In sharp contrast is the case of David Lawrence, former governor of Pennsylvania. He was the man who nominated Lyndon Johnson for Vice-President at the Democratic convention that chose John F. Kennedy as its presidential nominee.

On the evening of November 4, 1966, ex-Governor Lawrence was the principal speaker at a Democratic rally in Pittsburgh. In the middle of his speech his face turned gray and his forehead became clammy. He was gasping for breath and seemed to be struggling to utter a few more words. Then while some two thousand spectators watched in frozen silence, he collapsed to the floor.

The people who watched him with so much horror were helpless in the face of death until Karen McGuire, a nurse of Ohio Valley General Hospital, recognizing the deadly symptoms, rushed to the podium and began applying mouth-to-mouth resuscitation. Several of the governor's political friends also rallied to his side, and one of them began compressing the governor's chest in the hope of restarting circulation.

Minutes later police rushed into the auditorium with a stretcher. The former governor was taken to a waiting ambulance that sped to the emergency room at the University-Presbyterian Hospital. When word of the ex-governor's sudden collapse reached the hospital, some of the city's most eminent physicians quickly gathered to give him the care he would need.

But when Mr. Lawrence was carried into the emergency room, doctors could find no heartbeat, nor was he breathing. The last rites were administered by Father Thomas Ferris even as the team of doctors set into action the techniques that might revive the stricken heart. Cardiac resuscitation was started immediately. As the medical team worked to restart the heart, oxygenation of the patient's brain was instituted, for this is the critical area that must always be protected.

Dr. Campbell Moses, Medical Director of the American Heart Association, for twenty years personal physician to Mr. Lawrence, issued a statement to members of the press who crowded the door of the emergency room: "There is no heart action. The electrocardiogram shows no activity." However, Dr. Moses assured the press, the former governor had not suffered a heart attack. "It was a heart stoppage. He is not biologically dead. He is clinically dead."

By 9:45 the governor's heartbeat had been restored. He suffered another cardiac arrest later and again the beat was brought back. At 3 a.m. Dr. Moses reported to the press: "There is no evidence of heart damage. His heartbeat is remarkably strong."

At 5 A.M. the governor went into convulsions. This was the first indication that his brain had been damaged. It was then that doctors, checking back, wondered how long Mr. Lawrence had been deprived of oxygen. The ambulance ride that brought him to the hospital had taken ten minutes. No resuscitation was given during this time. Nor could the doctors ascertain how long before resuscitation was started from the time the governor had collapsed. But it was evidently long enough so that in the interim between his collapse and his arrival at the hospital his brain was forever shattered.

The next press report given by Dr. Moses was outspoken: "If it had been known immediately when the governor was brought into the emergency room he had been without oxygen for more than five or six minutes resuscitation procedures would not have been started because we would have known that his brain was gone and it was totally useless to bring him back. Death is inevitable."

Dr. Moses explained that an encephalogram taken after the convulsions showed severe brain damage, and added: "His entire brain is involved. The governor has no conscious appreciation of anything. He is dying not from heart failure, but from brain damage incurred when his heart stopped. There is no chance of recovery."

Because the governor's condition raised ethical and moral questions as well as medical, Dr. Moses consulted with Bishop John J. Wright of the Pittsburgh Catholic Diocese. Dr. Moses later told the press: "The Bishop understands our problem. It was agreed that we might continue all 'ordinary means' to preserve the former governor's life—but that we would not resort to extraordinary means. If his brain had not been injured, doctors would have gone to any lengths to maintain Mr. Lawrence's life." (It is possible to keep a dying patient alive indefinitely by connecting him to a machine that provides oxygen and circulation. When the respirator is cut off, the patient usually dies

within a few minutes. Such extraordinary therapy has been used
for organ transplants, where it is vital that the organ to be trans-
planted stay alive until the time has come to remove it.)

The governor, who had always been an exceptionally
healthy man, showed extraordinary vigor even in dying. In a
medical bulletin issued at University-Presbyterian Hospital on
November 7, three days after the heart stoppage, Dr. Moses
revealed that Mr. Lawrence "is now breathing without any assistance. The part of Mr. Lawrence's brain which controls his
breathing has recovered its function through this man's amazing
vitality. His clinging to life is not his conscious will—that is
gone—it is simply his vitality."

The doctor then added: "This does not mean—and I repeat
—this does not mean he has any chance of recovering. It is still
a hopeless case."

Mr. Lawrence died on November 21, 1966, seventeen days
after his first heart stoppage.

In most instances, the first person to arrive at the scene of
an accident is a layman. This makes it imperative that the public
learn the basic resuscitative techniques—external heart massage
and mouth-to-mouth breathing—which require no medical
knowledge whatsoever and can easily be mastered by any man,
woman, or teen-ager.

In Australia, for example, where the teaching of resuscitation starts with small school children and is made available to
every able-bodied person in the country, officials and doctors
have found that well-trained laymen can turn in a superb job
when resuscitation is needed to save a life.

At an international symposium on resuscitation, held at the
first European Congress of Anesthesiology in Vienna in 1963,
a representative of the Royal Life-Saving Society of Melbourne,
Australia, told the gathering of distinguished doctors:

You must reevaluate the knowledge of the layman. You
put him too far down the scale of intelligence. In some aspects

of livesaving, a layman who has had training could actually give you lessons concerning resuscitation.

We in Australia have special instructional units which teach the general public, beginning at the age of eight years. The people are taught mouth-to-mouth and mouth-to-nose ventilation, closed chest massage, and mouth-to-nose in water rescues. The grade of instruction is adapted to the average of the group. The more advanced the group, the more knowledge they are given.

The rate of sudden death in Australia has fallen markedly, even though the adult victim of unanticipated death has only four minutes' grace. This time element makes the role of the rescuer very significant. Used correctly, the new techniques can buy time for the victim by extending the state of clinical death for as long as two hours. While the mouth-to-mouth breathing and external heart massage continues, he remains alive. The critical maintenance of circulation and ventilation of the lungs protects the vital centers of the body, the most important of which are the brain and the heart. Both need inordinate amounts of oxygen. Without oxygen the tissues of the brain begin to die within minutes.

While it is obviously impossible in most cases of unexpected death to get a doctor to the scene within those first crucial minutes, resuscitative efforts immediately initiated by a layman allow bystanders to reach a doctor, to summon an ambulance, and to arrange for admittance to a hospital where the victim can receive the definitive care that will enable him to go on living.

The chances of a good outcome for the victim of sudden death is between 80 and 90 percent when resuscitation is started immediately and continued with vigorous persistence. It drops sharply to 10 percent if more than four or five minutes have passed.

So miraculously effective are these techniques that authorities state that resuscitation now offers the greatest immediate possibility of prolonging life. They predict that its widespread application would save more lives than would the appearance of a new and infallible cure for cancer.

Yet every day thousands of people throughout the United States, who might otherwise lead healthy, useful lives for many years if they received help in time, die—and are permitted to stay dead. Sudden death strikes everywhere—at a passenger in the automobile taking people on a holiday; it hovers near the swimming pool or beach; it is a frequent visitor at the playground where children find release for their energies. Sudden death is no stranger to the business office, the golf course, the crowded thoroughfare, the quiet home. It often comes when least expected, bringing tragedy and heartbreak.

Who can be resuscitated? A large percentage of those who die on any day. This includes those who succumb in a violent accident entailing massive loss of blood, in complex surgical operations, in childbirth, as well as victims of drowning or patients suffering from emphysema, pneumonia, asthma and other acute illnesses who seem to be recovering—but instead abruptly die. And, above all, many victims of heart disease.

That resuscitation techniques work is an accepted medical fact. Thousands who are alive today have been clinically dead. However, the child who succumbs to drowning, or the person critically injured in an accident, has a far better chance of being revived than the person who has been ill for a long time. Given help in time, the hearts of these victims have enough good, sound muscle to keep going for years. Recovery is no more hazardous than from any other illness. Most people who are brought back from clinical death suffer no physical aftereffects of any kind, and remain well and active for the rest of their life span.

How long can a brain survive without oxygen?

The fearful question "Will he be a vegetable?" haunts many a doctor and stays the hands and hearts of many a would-be Samaritan. It presents an agonizing dilemma—to resuscitate or not. The four-minute rule which is often used to designate the limit wherein resuscitation should take place after clinical death is easy to remember but is not always correct. For though prolonged lack of oxygen causes permanent damage, the meaning of the word "prolonged" varies widely in each case. Both the degree of hypoxia—lack of oxygen—and the tolerance of the patient are difficult to guess and no estimate in minutes can possibly be given say many doctors. Ideally, resuscitation should start instantly, for the victim's chances are always increased if he gets immediate help.

But many of the doctors most active in resuscitation believe firmly in giving the victim of sudden death every possible chance. Dr. James Jude says, "In the case of a border-line question as to the time of clinical death, it is always best to attempt resuscitation."

That a person on first recovering consciousness is confused does not mean that he has necessarily suffered permanent damage. The brain is slow to heal. In time, the patient can fully regain his capacities.

The fear that a person whose brain has been damaged by lack of oxygen might live on as a vegetable for years is not founded on fact. Medical experts in the art of resuscitation say that almost always the victim of brain damage dies within a few days.

Dr. Peter Safar, professor of anesthesiology and department chairman at the University-Presbyterian Hospital in Pittsburgh, feels that "anyone found in acute respiratory distress who is not known to be in terminal stages of an incurable disease should be considered savable and treated promptly with complete resuscitative effort."

Ideally everyone should know the methods that will help to save a human life, but doctors stress that knowledge of resuscitative techniques is urgently important to the relatives of a person suffering from a heart ailment and for the parents of small children. Accidents—choking, drowning, electrocution, swallowing poison, hazardous falls—take a dreadful toll of the lives of young children. Countless numbers of them could be saved if they received prompt help.

Many doctors have made independent efforts to teach mouth-to-mouth breathing and heart massage to the families of heart patients who may find it difficult to secure emergency help within the three to five crucial minutes.

Among the first such trainees was a middle-aged man who discovered his wife on the floor, crumpled in clinical death from a heart attack. Finding no signs of life in her, he began performing resuscitation. He had been taught that if he was alone he must give two or three quick mouth-to-mouth deep breaths, then alternate with fifteen heart manipulations. He continued this regimen, working steadily until his wife began breathing on her own. Then he was able to rouse a neighbor who drove them to the hospital while the husband continued his manipulations. His wife was saved.

Resuscitation can take place at any age. While doctors warn that people dying of an incurable disease such as cancer or those who have suffered severe brain damage should not be resuscitated, age has little to do with whether a person can make a good comeback. Dr. Safar resuscitated a woman of ninety-five who is now happily enjoying the company of her grandchildren and great-grandchildren.

Yet, despite the fact that there is available today the knowledge of resuscitation techniques that may one day prove important to every man and woman in America, there is in the United States no widespread movement to acquaint the public with the new and simple methods of saving a life—methods with which *anyone* can save a life.

In a country noted for its scientific power and progress, for its generous aid to countries in need, it seems ironic that thousands of young and vital citizens are permitted to pass away because no concentrated effort has been made to salvage lives.

An elderly man suffering from pneumonia is given every care. The family doctor is called, or a specialist may be consulted. Hospitalization is arranged by the physician in charge.

But when a forty-year-old man suddenly drops dead from heart stoppage, a two-year-old child chokes to death on a piece of candy or a teen-ager races his motorcycle into a stone wall— they are allowed to die. For when sudden death strikes, confusion, panic, apathy, and carelessness often dominate the scene and a life is lost by default.

3.

ASPHYXIA—THE INVISIBLE STRANGLER

In a restaurant in Yonkers, New York, Margaret W., a seventeen-year-old girl, suddenly rose from her table, clutched at her chest and collapsed to the floor. When a doctor arrived, he pronounced her dead of a heart attack. Two days later the medical examiner reported that she had actually been the victim of a tragic and avoidable accident. A piece of meat had choked her to death. If only it had been removed in time and artificial respiration applied, she would have lived.

In a Boston drugstore, a little girl ordered a chocolate soda. While the clerk prepared it, she played with a red balloon. When her soda arrived, the child began to sip it. Suddenly she fell from the stool. The clerk ran to her side and found to his horror that she was dead. A doctor arrived fifteen minutes later but it was too late for him to help her. She had passed into biological death. An autopsy established the fact that she had sucked in the balloon with her soda. Within seconds it had sealed tight her air passage. The child did not have time to cough or cry out before she lost consciousness and almost immediately smothered to death.

Life began, according to the biblical allegory, when the Lord breathed into a lump of clay. Even two thousand years ago people recognized that breath is the first requirement of life. Man can survive without food for several weeks; without water for three or four days; but without air only three or four minutes. Lack of breath—medically known as asphyxia—causes fifty thousand deaths in this country each year. Almost all of these can easily be reversed if those surrounding the victim are able to recognize the signs and know the simple procedures that must be followed to return the breath of life.

It's when death by choking or strangulation in a single moment overtakes an otherwise healthy person that it is especially shattering. It can happen in the midst of a gay party, at a quiet family meal, a children's picnic. This type of accident often befalls the middle-aged who wear dentures—especially if they have had a couple of drinks and are careless in chewing—a child engrossed in play while eating, a person suffering from a cold who may have difficulty swallowing a large morsel of food, or someone laughing and talking while in the process of eating.

Even though surrounded by relatives or friends, they die within minutes because few people recognize that choking can lead to a painful and terrifying death. Often it mimics the symptoms of a heart attack. There is the swift pallor turning to cyanosis (the skin turns blue from lack of oxygen), the cessation of breathing, the loss of pulse.

If a new germ were to appear, decimating the lives of men, women, and children as does asphyxia, the public would clamor for relief. But because asphyxia seems like a fate that is part of human destiny, people accept the needless deaths without a murmur. Yet only a little knowledge—knowledge that can often be learned in minutes—may save the life of a man, woman, or child choking to death.

A tragic example of how quickly asphyxia can kill was demonstrated by the death of Mrs. Joan Patricia Skakel, the sister-in-law of Mrs. Ethel Kennedy. On a warm evening in May, 1967, Mrs. Skakel gave a dinner party at her home in Greenwich, Connecticut. The guests of the thirty-nine-year-old hostess were old friends. It was one of the first parties she had given since her husband, George Skakel, Jr., had crashed in a small airplane seven months earlier.

The main course served at the dinner was shishkebab—

skewered lamb. Abruptly, Mrs. Skakel, who had been talking animatedly, began to cough. Someone leaned over and gave her a slap on the back. Someone else offered her a glass of water and solicitous queries and advice came from all sides. "Are you all right?" "Try swallowing" and "Drink some water" were among the suggestions.

But the coughing became worse and Mrs. Skakel began to gag and gasp for breath. Terribly embarrassed but unable to excuse herself she gestured with her hands as she fled to the bathroom. The party went on. No one realized the seriousness of her discomfort. After a considerable time had elapsed and she had not returned, one of the guests went to see if she could offer help. She found Mrs. Skakel collapsed on the bathroom floor. She was pronounced dead on arrival at Greenwich Hospital. Mrs. Skakel had died of strangulation when a piece of meat lodged in her throat.

The death of Mrs. Skakel was one more of the tragedies that could have been avoided if the public knew more about the subject of asphyxia. Had any of the guests at the party realized the gravity of the situation and known just what to do, her life could have been saved.

Mrs. Skakel should have been allowed to cough without interruption. For when a piece of meat, or some other aspirated object lodges in the larynx, it frequently causes a violent spasm which, in turn, causes choking. When the spasm relaxes, the person is often able to cough up the object that is causing the distress. But the party atmosphere, the slap on the back, the friends who kept asking if she wanted a drink and if she was all right, only made matters worse. By running from the table and secluding herself in the bathroom, Mrs. Skakel signed her death warrant.

Even after she had collapsed there would still have been a chance to save her life by administering mouth-to-mouth resuscitation, which would have kept her in clinical death until a doctor was summoned. As a person loses consciousness, muscle tone is lost. This makes mouth-to-mouth breathing more effective since it is easier for air to get through to the lungs, where it is desperately needed. But Mrs. Skakel was beyond help when her friends finally came looking for her.

Equally tragic was the death of Sherwood Anderson, one of America's most illustrious writers. Anderson was at the height of his fame in 1940 when he was sent as an American envoy of good will to South America. An ironic victim of peripheral literary activities, he choked to death on a toothpick in a canape at a literary cocktail party.

Many industries today teach resuscitation techniques to all their employees—a program that has paid off in lives saved time and time again. But when the knowledge of resuscitation helps to save the life of one's own child, it becomes the most important lesson one can ever learn.

When William McTeer took the course in resuscitation at Outside Plan Construction Department classes in Ossining, New York, he didn't dream that within a few days his new knowledge would save the life of his twenty-two-month-old daughter, Lorie Anne. The little girl, seated in a high chair, was eating her lunch when suddenly she choked on a piece of French toast. Mr. McTeer, who fortunately was home, recalls that in a matter of seconds, she turned blue, her eyes rolled up into her head, her body became limp and her head, arms, and legs began to twitch.

Frantically McTeer worked to dislodge the morsel, hoping thus to revive her. When his efforts failed, he quickly put her on the table and started mouth-to-mouth breathing. Although Lorie Anne's chest expanded, showing she was getting oxygen, she remained unconscious.

Most people do not realize that mouth-to-mouth breathing often dislodges obstructions, especially if the victim is a child. An adult's breath blown into a child's throat is always powerful; it can clear the passage as well as supply life-saving oxygen.

Mr. McTeer carried Lorie Anne out to the car. His wife, who had been taught how to apply rescue breathing by Mr. McTeer, continued resuscitation while he drove the twelve miles to the nearest hospital. There doctors told the McTeers that, although Lorie Anne was in shock, the morsel of food had been dislodged by the mouth-to-mouth breathing. Her parents had saved her life.

Respiratory illness in young children may result in choking or strangling. It can be a temporary lack of oxygen that brings on asphyxia, regurgitated food that obstructs the windpipe, or edema (swelling) that causes acute congestion and results in smothering. These situations can be reversed if resuscitation is given quickly.

That even a child can competently save a life if he has had proper instruction was proven recently in Larchmont, New York, where members of the sixth grade of the Chatsworth Avenue grammar school are taught the basic techniques of resuscitation. All of the eleven- and twelve-year-olds learned to do rescue breathing. Little did anyone realize how important this lesson would soon prove.

It was only a day after the class demonstration that two of the pupils had a chance to show how prepared they were to come to the rescue of anyone in trouble. Gino Del Guercio was in the yard playing when he heard a splash—his twenty-month-old sister had fallen into the goldfish pool. With his mother screaming and other members of the family in panic, Gino took charge. Diving in, he rescued his little sister. But when he brought her out of the water he discovered that she was not breathing.

Without waiting a second, he placed her on the ground and began doing mouth-to-mouth breathing. While other members of the family stood immobile, frantic with terror, Gino continued breathing for the little girl. After a few minutes the child moved, and uttered a sharp cry. Soon the little girl was herself again, thanks to the quick thinking of her older brother, who had learned his lesson well.

When Mike McGarey, also a member of the sixth grade class, got home from school he was so proud of his new accomplishment that he immediately demonstrated how it was done.

His older brother, fourteen-year-old Charles, watched carefully and asked a number of questions to make sure he was getting it right.

That same evening their younger brother, three-year-old Chris, was put to bed immediately after supper. When Mrs. McGarey went in to check on him she found the little boy rigid and blue and no longer breathing. She screamed, "Get a doctor! Quick!"

While Mike raced to the phone, Charles ran into Chris's bedroom. He placed the small boy on the floor and, following carefully the directions Mike had given, began blowing air into the three-year-old's lungs. Even before the doctor arrived, Chris had begun to breathe though he was still in difficulty.

Chris had eaten hamburger for supper. Shortly after he fell asleep he regurgitated the food, which choked off his breath. Charles's quick thinking saved his life for it supplied him with much needed oxygen until he could be taken to a hospital and given further treatment.

John J. Madey, principal of the Chatsworth School, told the whole class about the quick thinking and heroic efforts of their two classmates who had made such good use of their knowledge. "Michelle and Chris wouldn't have revived but for the know-how of their brothers," he told them.

A case of successful resuscitation recently performed by a young mother showed such a valiant spirit and clear thinking it brought salutes of admiration from skilled surgeons.

Parents who are terrified at the thought of putting their fingers down the throat of a child who is choking on a morsel of food or who shudder at learning to do mouth-to-mouth resuscitation, though no possible harm can possibly come from it, should draw inspiration from the courage displayed by this mother.

Mrs. R., who for many years was an efficient operating room nurse, was fixing lunch for her family when she heard her six-year-old daughter, Betsy, scream in pain. Rushing out into the yard, where the girl had been playing, Mrs. R. discovered Betsy had been stung by a bee. Allergic to the bee venom, Betsy was lying on the ground unconscious when the mother reached her. Swelling of the larynx had completely blocked Betsy's breathing and was choking the child as surely as if a killer had placed his hands around her throat.

Gathering Betsy up in her arms, the mother raced back to the kitchen where she placed the child, now clinically dead, on the kitchen table. She knew there was no time to wait for a doctor or an ambulance. If the child was to live she must have immediate help. Because of the swelling in the throat, mouth-to-mouth breathing would be useless since the air would not be able to reach the lungs. Her years in the operating room told Mrs. R. what was needed—a tracheotomy, an operation in which an opening is made in the throat where a tube for oxygenation can be inserted. This operation has many dangers and is one that doctors often hesitate to undertake.

But the mother, who knew well the difficulties inherent in the operation, felt she had no choice. Betsy's lungs now were cut off from any source of oxygen.

Mrs. R. had seen the operation performed many times, always by a surgeon with proper tools and with meticulous attention to sterilization. But there was no time to worry about niceties. Quickly she began to improvise. An old fountain pen was dismantled. The barrel had two holes and she washed it thoroughly in hot water.

Fear almost paralyzed her as she went about making her preparations. What if she made a mistake? But she couldn't let herself swim in that sea. Her child was already clinically dead. And another part of her brain told her, "If I can give her oxygen she will survive. There will be time to call a doctor, to get her to a hospital for the urgent care she needs—the antibiotics, the vital transfusions if she loses too much blood."

But the next step was almost her undoing. With a kitchen knife in her hand she thought for a moment she'd black out—she couldn't cut into that small, vulnerable throat. But she knew it was imperative to do so. If she fainted or panicked, she would be failing her child.

Carefully she explored the throat, found the exact spot where she had seen surgeons make the incision—a spot that would bypass the swelling and permit air to enter the lungs. Quickly she made the incision and pushed in the fountain pen barrel. Once properly inserted it was a fair substitute for the tracheal tube she had seen used in hospitals. She began to blow air into one of the holes and watched as Betsy's small chest began to move. Through the improvised tracheal tube the life-saving air moved in and out.

Mrs. R. continued resuscitation while a neighbor who had heard her screams telephoned for an ambulance. Betsy, with her mother still breathing for her, was taken to the hospital. Doctors were astonished at the professional job. She had observed well, and because she had her child made a perfect recovery.

Fortunately, few cases require such extreme action. Certainly this is not recommended as a form of resuscitation to be attempted by the average layman. Mrs. R. had the advantage of knowing how the operation was performed. In the hands of a totally untrained person, a tracheotomy would result in instant death.

Although most babies are born in hospitals, occasionally one puts in an early and unexpected appearance. At such times the policeman, who has had good training in emergency care, can perform with skill and knowledge.

Patrolman Anthony Cuomo saved a life because, in addition to his knowledge of obstetrics, he had received training in resuscitation techniques. Accompanied by his partner, Patrolman Charles Temnski, Cuomo found twenty-three-year-old Mrs. Alice Ward alone in her Brooklyn apartment in labor.

The father of two, Patrolman Cuomo was an old hand at helping babies into the world—he had a score of seventeen births —and he immediately took over. Quietly calming Mrs. Ward, he helped her deliver a five-pound-three-ounce boy. He was at his patrol car checking on the progress of an ambulance he had ordered for the mother and her newborn son, when he heard Temnski shout from the Ward apartment.

He hurried back and discovered his work was only half done. Mrs. Ward was having twins. The second delivery was also a boy of five pounds five ounces. But he was blue and not breathing. Cuomo quickly started mouth-to-mouth resuscitation. By the time the ambulance attendant from Wyckoff Hospital arrived with the oxygen tank, the baby was crying lustily.

At the same time, in a New York hospital where every care should be expected, a young woman was delivered of a blue, flaccid baby. The attending obstetrician, busy with the mother, handed the infant to an assistant for resuscitation. Uncertain as to what to do, the young intern simply held the limp child. When the obstetrician spoke sharply to him, pointing out there was no time to lose, the intern began "tubbing" the baby—an old-fashioned and ineffective method in which the infant is immersed in warm then in cold water to stimulate breathing.

Yet only a few feet away was the life-saving oxygen that the child needed. Making sure the mother was safe, the obstetrician took over. Inserting a tube into the baby's windpipe, he sucked out the mucus obstructing it. He then inserted another tube leading to a tank holding a mixture of oxygen and carbon dioxide. The oxygen sustained the baby's life. The carbon dioxide acted as a stimulant to start the infant breathing. Within a few minutes, the baby had turned from blue to pink and was giving its first cry.

Countless other babies are not so lucky. The annual death rate of newborn babies in America is a shocking 200,000!

Dr. E. M. Papper, former director of Anesthesiology Service at Presbyterian Hospital in New York, a noted authority in his field, states that restoring breathing is the first movement of resuscitation and one that must be quickly attended to when a baby arrives into the world. For few events are so perilous as a baby's struggle for his first breath. From a passive recipient of oxygen dissolved in his mother's blood, he must make the transition to a detached and squalling human being, gulping in the fresh air of the outside world. And he must accomplish this shift within a very few minutes or suffer terrible consequences.

Many babies don't have a chance to live because they are unable to make the transition. Of all the infants who die in the first twenty-four hours of their lives—and the annual deaths of newborn babies in New York City alone is 5,500—it is estimated that about one-fifth die of asphyxia—lack of oxygen. These babies do not cry or thrash about. They lie silently, for the baby born limp, blue, or flaccid needs oxygen just as much as the man who collapses suddenly with a heart attack, the drowning boy who is pulled out of a swimming pool, or the child who is asphyxiated when he locks himself in an old icebox. Yet few women expecting babies check the qualifications of their obstetrician, make sure a trained anesthetist will be available, and that the hospital in which the birth of the baby will take place has modern equipment. They fail to realize that whether the child is stillborn or, more disastrous, born with a damaged brain, may depend entirely on the quality of the care they receive.

There are four and a half million babies delivered in hospitals each year and many more in homes. Because of the shortage of doctors and nurses, many babies enter the world without proper obstetrical or anesthesiological care, says Dr. Papper. He points out that unfortunately obstetrical anesthesia, which involves young lives, has taken second place to surgical anesthesia.

Anyone needing surgery, no matter how minor, is apt to be provided with a trained anesthesiologist. For the surgeon recognizes that his reputation is at stake if the anesthetist bungles. An error in anesthetic management which invariably leads to asphyxia is the primary or contributing factor in more than 20 percent of the ten thousand surgical deaths per year. Experts in the field say unequivocally that these deaths in the final analysis are due to inadequate resuscitation.

Because deliveries are unscheduled, a young mother may be cared for by an intern incapable of handling emergencies should they arise. If the baby had the umbilical cord wrapped around his throat, if the mother had a difficult labor and required a large quantity of drugs, or if she suffered from low blood pressure during the pregnancy, the newborn baby desperately needs help. When doctors have had good training, the newborn is always given resuscitation immediately. Too often, however, little or nothing is done for the newcomer and he may slip away without uttering a cry of protest.

Just how bad is the situation is reflected in the following statistics: *50 percent of births in the nation are unattended by personnel trained in anesthesia and fewer than 1 percent of the nation's 649 maternity hospitals provide twenty-four-hour anesthesia service, although half of the deliveries occur at night.*

So little thought and time has been given to resuscitation in this country that many physicians do not even recognize asphyxia when it occurs in a patient they are treating. In a New York hospital, because no anesthetist was available, a young woman received local anesthesia from her obstetrician when she went into labor. The doctor, unfamiliar with dosage, gave her too much sedation. Suddenly the woman went into convulsions. The doctor did not realize she was reacting to the drug and urgently needed oxygen. He thought she was suffering from eclampsia—a severe type of toxemia that can occur during pregnancy—and gave her more sedation. When the woman did not respond and it was obvious she was in great danger, he put through a call for an anesthetist. The woman died before help arrived.

Nor is this an isolated case. Just how common are these fully preventable deaths was recently revealed by a questionnaire that was circulated among seventy-five doctors in New York City. The answers disclosed that seven of the queried doctors stood helplessly by while their patients went into what they termed "sudden and inexplicable death" after they had administered anesthetics or antitoxins.

Dr. Papper urges that every medical student receive training in anesthesiology, the course wherein the essentials of proper medical resuscitation are taught. For, no matter in what field he plans to specialize, every doctor should be skilled in the art of returning the breath of life.

A special conference on infant mortality sponsored by the AMA Committee on Maternal and Child Care pointed out that there are 24.2 deaths per 1,000 births. To improve the survival chances of newborn infants, the committee urged that present know-how in the care of premature infants be extended to hospitals throughout the country and that all anesthetists and obstetricians familarize themselves with the newest methods of resuscitation.

Hypoxia, which means a deficit of oxygen, has become more common since a variety of new drugs came into use. The wide assortment of sleeping pills used by countless thousands of Americans is a growing danger. Though an overdose of these pills induces a slower death, in the end asphyxia takes over. The drugs commonly used to induce sleep tend to slow up breathing, and when taken to excess will paralyze the controlling center of respiration in the brain. However, the victims found early enough usually respond to resuscitation.

In Malibu, California, on November 9, 1967, actress Jennifer Jones took an overdose of sleeping pills, then phoned her doctor from a pay station to bid him good-bye. Alarmed, he quickly notified the police who were able to trace the call. A clerk at a motel told them Miss Jones had checked in the night before using the name of Phyllis Walker. (She was born Phyllis Isley in Tulsa, Oklahoma, and was married to the late actor Robert Walker before marrying David O. Selznick.) The clerk said that the actress went to a telephone booth a block away when she was told there was no phone in her room.

Checking further the police found Miss Jones's sports car, its lights still on, parked at the top of a four-hundred-foot cliff. Wearing a white shirt and tan slacks the Oscar-winning actress lay unconscious on the rock-strewn base of the cliff as the surf washed over her.

Sergeant Eldon Loken, one of those who found the actress,

later said: "I thought she was dead." He immediately started mouth-to-mouth resuscitation. "I held my flashlight to her face so I could see any response. She was very quiet. Then her breath started to come."

The actress was rushed to an emergency hospital where her stomach was pumped. Traces of seconal and evidence that she had been drinking some sort of wine were found. Investigators said an empty champagne bottle was in her car.

Miss Jones was transferred to the Intensive Care Unit at Mount Sinai Hospital in Los Angeles. She remained unconscious for six hours. But she eventually made a complete recovery.

Although no reason for the attempted suicide was ever given, Miss Jones called her doctor only an hour after she learned that Charles Bickford, the leading actor in her greatest film, *The Song of Bernadette*, had died suddenly of a heart attack.

Miss Jones, who disliked publicity, rarely appeared in public after her marriage to movie tycoon Selznick. The man who made *Gone With the Wind* and who was instrumental in making Miss Jones one of the outstanding movie stars of her time died in 1965. Miss Jones is the mother of three children—two grown sons by Walker and a daughter, Mary Jennifer, by Selznick.

Almost at the same time that Miss Jones was undergoing her ordeal, a thirty-two-year-old woman left her home in Los Angeles and registered at a small hotel. A quarrel with her husband had precipitated her frantic departure from home. Alone in her hotel room she swallowed forty sleeping pills—a powerful dose which would guarantee death. Twenty-four hours later the woman was discovered by a maid. It looked hopeless since so long a time had elapsed. But fortunately the doctor who arrived within minutes was an expert in treating asphyxia. He immediately inserted a plastic tube in her throat attached to a rubber bag which provided oxygen directly to her lungs. He continued resuscitation in the ambulance that took her to a hospital where an oxygen tank was placed beside her bed. For 144 hours—six full days—while she remained in a coma, oxygen was poured into her lungs and artificial respiration continued. The case that looked hopeless had a happy ending. When the woman recovered consciousness, she was reconciled with her husband. With the help of psychotherapy, the couple was able to resume life on a happier basis.

Modern resuscitation has also been effective when used on suicide victims of hanging. If cut down quickly enough and given mouth-to-mouth resuscitation they can be brought back to life.

The new resuscitative techniques have also saved lives of our growing number of drug addicts. Dr. Helene Mayer, who has done extensive work with addicted children, says that our terrible death rate would be even greater if most addicts were not knowledgeable about resuscitation. When an addict has taken an overdose he is often saved by a buddy who immediately does mouth-to-mouth breathing, providing the desperately needed oxygen.

Says Dr. Mayer: "Most of the addicts, even the very young children, know this is their only hope of turning back death. They all know how to do it effectively. Unfortunately an addict is often alone when taking drugs and there is no one to help him when he gets into difficulties."

Almost every person who loses consciousness for any reason whatever is a potential victim of asphyxia and a potential beneficiary of resuscitation properly administered. For the unconscious person—whether he is the victim of gas poisoning, smoke, drugs, a heart attack, or accidental injury—generally loses the ability to swallow or cough. If something lodges in his respiratory tract, even something as seemingly insignificant as a small clot of phlegm, he may choke to death unless he has proper treatment immediately. In the tragic Coconut Grove disaster in 1942, 491 people died when the Boston nightclub caught fire. But a number of the bodies showed no traces of burns. Had these victims of asphyxia received modern resuscitation many of them could have been saved.

Many deaths listed as resulting from asthma, pneumonia, convulsions, epileptic seizures, and heart failure can often be reversed if there is someone present to resuscitate the patient. All of them desperately need oxygen.

Mr. Harold Bassett, director of First Aid of the American Red Cross in greater New York, states that countless deaths attributed to heart attack are, in reality, due to strangulation. Everyone knows of cases where a person suddenly collapsed in what appeared to be a typical heart attack after eating a large meal. Mr. Bassett says that often the collapse is caused by food regurgitating and blocking the air passage. The victim succumbs unless help is available. By using two fingers wrapped in a clean handkerchief to quickly clear the passageway and immediately starting mouth-to-mouth breathing, the process of death can be reversed.

Tragically, small children are often the victims of the strangler. The National Safety Council lists foreign bodies as the leading cause of home accidental deaths among children under five years of age. In fact, inhalation and ingestion of food and foreign objects kill more children than does polio, tuberculosis, and five other major childhood diseases combined.

The toddler is old enough to get into trouble but too young to know better. Often it is carelessness and lack of knowledge on the part of parents that is responsible when disaster overtakes them.

Few people realize that choking and gagging have deadly implications. Fortunately not all foreign objects taken into the mouth end in strangulation and death. Often the object is swallowed. But this does not mean it can be forgotten. On the contrary, the longer it remains inside the body the more harm it is likely to do.

There have been many cases where people have endured severe illness for years as a result of swallowing a foreign object. Only when it was removed from some vital part of their body was there relief. But in some cases when too much time has elapsed incalculable damage is done.

Recently a mother in Chicago noticed that her little girl, just one year old, was having difficulty swallowing. The child took her food slowly and it gurgled on the way down. Alarmed, the mother took the child to a doctor. X rays clearly revealed part of the story: metal obstruction in the esophagus. By the time the surgeon had finished exploring the child's throat he had removed one ball bearing, one washer, a piece of wood, several wads of paper, a flake of metal, and a strip of pink plastic.

The surgeon in this case was Dr. Paul N. Hollinger, attending broncho-esophagologist at Children's Memorial Hospital in Chicago. The odd collection of objects that he found in the little girl's throat was no surprise to him. It merely confirmed what he has been telling parents for years: "If given a chance youngsters will swallow anything."

During the last thirty years, Dr. Hollinger and his associates have removed about five thousand dangerous objects from the throats, lungs, and intestines of children. They included, among other things, small coins, safety pins, melon seeds, peanuts, popcorn kernels, a bolt, a red crayon, a doll's eye, a .22-caliber bullet, a Goldwater button, and in one instance a turtle!

Safely removed, these oddities have a certain humor. But many of the objects lodged in a child's body are grimly unfunny.

"It is true," says Dr. Hollinger, "that many swallowed objects pass harmlessly through a child's system. But others get stuck in the esophagus or intestines—or worse, go down the 'wrong way' and are sucked into the windpipe or lungs."

The possible results are infection, respiratory difficulties, a blockage of airways that can cause asphyxiation and, in the case of sharp objects, a puncture of the membranes with serious or even fatal hemorrhaging.

Doctors urge that if a child has had a choking incident, even though he seems to recover, parents should arrange to have him thoroughly examined by a physician.

The Red Cross lists the following do's and don'ts:

Keep small objects such as pins, buttons, coins, and jewelry out of reach of children. Only sturdy toys without small parts that might become detached should be provided for play.

Do not give small children food such as peanuts, popcorn, food containing nuts (especially candy bars and cereal), raw vegetables, fruit with seeds, or unchopped meat.

Do not permit a child to run while eating.

Do not permit children under five to chew bubble gum. If swallowed, it may seal off the esophagus and cause strangulation.

Older children in the family group should be educated to the importance of preventive measures and should assist in the project of making potential foreign bodies unavailable.

For adults the Red Cross suggests:

Use extra care in preparing foods containing bones. Persons eating chicken sandwiches, salads, or soup do not expect to encounter foreign objects and frequently swallow small bones. When game birds are shot, pieces of bone and shotgun pellets may remain imbedded in the meat and can become foreign bodies if not removed when the meat is prepared.

Persons who wear dentures should keep them in good repair. The denture wearer should chew his food longer than he did when he had his natural teeth. Dentures should be removed at night unless otherwise advised by the dentist.

Holding pins, needles, nails, or similar objects in the mouth is dangerous practice for an adult and sets a bad example for a child.

When a choking accident does occur, keep calm and try to encourage the victim to cough up the object.

Don't distract him by showing alarm or asking questions.

Don't give him bread to propel the foreign body into the stomach. (This old-fashioned remedy is apt to make removal more difficult because of excessive gastric secretions.)

Don't slap him on the back. It might cause the person to cough the offending object back against the vocal cords, which would result in suffocation.

If the object cannot be dislodged by the victim's normal

mechanisms, rush the patient to a hospital or quickly phone for a doctor.

If the patient has collapsed, start emergency techniques immediately. Put hand under neck, thus throwing head back and opening wide the mouth. Start mouth-to-mouth breathing. This will keep him alive until medical help can be obtained.

4.
ACCIDENTS HAPPEN
TO THE YOUNG

Deaths by fire, deaths by drowning, deaths which outrace speed on the highway, and deaths caused by freak, seemingly unpredictable accidents added up to 113,169 in 1967—most of them involving young people.

Throughout the world accident as a cause of death is outranked only by cancer and cardiovascular disease. For young people—from ages one to thirty-seven—death by accident is at the top of the list. Teen-agers and young adults race souped-up cars, take reckless chances in the water, ski on hazardous mountains. And young men and women lead the list in fatalities caused by industrial accidents. As the labor supply has declined and production schedules increased, employers have been forced to hire more inexperienced personnel, which often means young people who have no training.

Accidents take more lives of children under five than all the children's diseases put together. We've conquered many of the killer diseases—polio, diphtheria, typhoid—that used to annihilate children. But swimming pools, automobiles, bicycles, poison—to mention a few of the hazards—have taken their place.

The accidental death of a child is always heartbreaking, but especially so when you realize that a child has a much longer span of time than an adult during which death can be reversed. While most doctors believe that the average adult has from three to five minutes before biological death sets in, a child stays in clinical death between eight and ten minutes. And there are case histories of critically injured children who were dead for as long as twenty-five minutes but who made excellent recoveries. For children are much less likely to have permanent neurological and psychological damage. Dr. Peter Safar, of Pittsburgh's University-Presbyterian Hospital, has found that even when the injury has been severe and unconsciousness has persisted for as long as a week the child often makes a complete recovery.

A dramatic case in which a young housewife survived more than twenty-one minutes of circulatory arrest may revise many of the calculations now prevalent on the survival time for adults.

On Saturday afternoon, July, 31, 1965, Mrs. Alexis Powell was thrown into the steering wheel when her car collided head-on with another vehicle. When she was brought into the emergency unit of San Francisco General Hospital minutes after the crash, she was unconscious and in shock, with signs of severe head injury, a crushed chest, and abdominal injuries. She had bled profusely and was immediately given a large volume of blood and intravenous fluids. Her condition stabilized through the hours of the morning.

But nineteen hours after the accident her condition suddenly became critical. She was being readied for an X ray when her blood pressure became nonexistent and only "distant" heart sounds were detectable.

The emergency was such that no time was lost in long preparation as she was rushed to the operating room.

"We quite literally threw her on the operating table and I slashed an incision," was the way Dr. Benson B. Roe, who headed the surgical team, described the urgent situation.

A record of less than ten minutes was set between the time when clinical death first appeared in the X ray department and when the patient was being operated on.

Dr. Roe, in describing the operation, said that though Mrs. Powell's heart was beating weakly, she was moribund. He had hardly started the operation when an overwhelming flood of blood filled the entire chest cavity and overflowed on both sides of the table in "immeasureable quantities." After six or eight minutes to clear the operating field with suction, Dr. Roe resorted to induced fibrillation. "I had to stop the heart," he explained. "I had no choice." The bold maneuver was thwarted by still another flood. Desperately but unsuccessfully the surgeons attempted to plug the wound.

There was only one thing left to do—shut off the blood supply of the entire body. There was no time to set up the heart-lung unit used when circulation must be curtailed. Mrs. Powell's heart stopped beating and no pulse was discernible.

As Dr. Roe repaired the damage to the heart—a matter of delicate suturing, perilous because of penetrating the adjacent aorta (a main artery)—he was fearful that if the girl lived, she would come out of the operation a mindless creature.

Before he cut off the circulation, Dr. Roe tried heart massage twice, for about ten seconds each time. "It was an awfully flabby, soft, and bloodless heart. I believe that by this time she was essentially bled out." He did not think it worthwhile to continue massaging.

According to the anesthesiologist's chart, there was virtually no circulation during a period of twenty-one minutes starting from the time when the chest was opened. Dr. Roe took about ten minutes to clear the field and another ten minutes after inducing fibrillation to repair the damaged heart and close the wound. The big veins were shut off for about seven minutes.

With circulation completely cut off and no oxygen feeding her brain, the chances of her coming out with her faculties intact seemed very slim, indeed. But within an hour of surgery, Mrs. Powell was awake and rational. Her surgeon described her condition as "zero neurological deficit."

Dr. Roe, who in retrospect feels the length of Mrs. Powell's circulatory arrest defies belief, is of the opinion that brain survival time is greatly underestimated. "It's my feeling—no, I'm actually convinced—that the brain can withstand arrested circulation for more than four minutes with complete, undamaged survival."

Dr. William F. Heer, vascular surgeon, agrees that the brain's capacity to recover from such insults may be underestimated, but he notes, "this is not a predictably reproducible phenomenon."

The California surgeons suggest some possibilities that might explain the survival after the long period without circulation. During the time when the copious flow of blood was uncontrolled, some four liters or more of cold bank blood were pumped into the patient's veins, which may have produced a mild hypothermia. And the massage may have provided just enough circulation.

"Obviously," Dr. Roe notes, "something must have happened to give some kind of circulation. But by usual criteria, the flow was virtually nonexistent."

In the more than fifty thousand annual highway accidents, injuries involving the head and thorax are the most common causes of death. Such injuries are often associated with respiratory distress. If given adequate resuscitation immediately, many of these victims of sudden death could live.

On a warm afternoon in June, 1968, two automobiles smashed into each other on a superhighway. State troopers were lifting three young boys and a girl out of the wreckage. Two white-coated interns waited.

The bodies were broken and covered with blood. All appeared to be dead. But fortunately these interns knew that in automobile accidents the cause of clinical death is not necessarily the result of injuries, grievous though they may be, but of escaping carbon monoxide inhaled by the unconscious victims. Questioned by the doctors, the troopers had ascertained that carbon monoxide was escaping from the wrecked cars. It was reasonable to hope that oxygen would revive the victims and give them a chance to fight for their lives under expert medical care.

It was too late for two of the boys, for the severe injuries incurred as the cars smashed head-on had already brought biological death. But the other boy and the girl had apparently lost consciousness and gone into clinical death as a result of the escaping gas. They responded to mouth-to-mouth breathing within a few minutes. Carefully placing them in the ambulance, the interns continued first aid until the hospital emergency room was reached where a team of experts took over. The young people's lives were saved.

Carbon monoxide, the second most common cause of death due to poisoning, is not always identified as the villain. Almost anyone recognizes carbon monoxide as the killer when he finds a locked car with a person slumped over the wheel. But in many cases, it is not even suspected because carbon monoxide rapidly leaves the bloodstream. Death is then attributed to something else or listed as "cause unknown."

Dr. Milton Helpern, Medical Examiner of New York City, recalls the case of a twenty-seven-year-old man who was found dead in his bed. Nearby lay his father in a comatose condition. An autopsy established the fact that the boy had died of carbon monoxide, but doctors at the hospital were unable to find any trace of the poison in the father's bloodstream though he was near death. Nor could investigators find the lethal poison in the apartment.

Not until they stopped on the first floor to talk to the landlord did they find the answer. It was bitter cold and the room was heated by an old-fashioned stove. The flue which reached up into the bedroom occupied by the father and son was defective. Sleeping soundly through the cold night, both men had inhaled the fumes. The father died several hours after he was taken to the hospital, thus marking up another score for the poison which has the characteristics of a sneak thief.

Dr. Helpern, investigating further, found that the mother had died a month earlier and that her death had been attributed to illness. Actually, she, too, had been a victim of the insidious poison that floated up from the apartment below.

Carbon monoxide, which primarily attacks the brain and the

heart, is all too common a cause for illness and death. While every effort should be made to eliminate the source, once a person is stricken he should receive immediate resuscitation. If caught early enough, oxygen and heart massage will revive the victim.

The fact that a layman can effectively use resuscitation techniques by following printed instructions was superbly demonstrated by Mrs. Lorrie Meyer who, with her husband, Ben, and their five young children, lives on a ranch in the remote regions of the Colorado mountains. Mrs. Meyer was just putting a cake in the oven when she heard a commotion in the yard. Running outside, she found her seven-year-old-son, Fritz, apparently dead, stretched out on the ground in front of their vintage car. The other children stood about screaming and crying. Her husband seemed frozen in a state of shock.

Fritz had ridden home with his father who is employed as a horse-trainer on the ranch. Jumping off and on the running board of the car, he opened and closed the gates of the paddocks. As he closed the last gate, instead of taking his place on the running board, he hopped up on the fender. Mr. Meyer, who had the motor going, was already in gear when Fritz started sliding. Before the father could apply the brakes, the left front wheel had passed over his son's chest.

Mrs. Meyer bent over her son. He wasn't breathing, nor could she detect any heartbeat. Yet the terrified mother remembered a life insurance advertisement she had pasted on her kitchen wall. It gave directions for mouth-to-mouth resuscitation. She had never actually studied the ad, but as she bent over her child's body, it was as if the directions were spelled out in front of her.

She placed a hand under the small boy's neck, which threw his head back and opened wide his mouth. She placed her other hand on his forehead, letting her thumb close off the nose. Taking a deep breath, she covered Fritz's mouth firmly with her own and exhaled. As she turned her head away in order to inhale she thought she saw a small movement of the chest. She continued breathing for her child. The movement of the boy's chest became pronounced.

Mr. Farnes, owner of the ranch, phoned ahead to the family doctor in Evergreen, then drove Mrs. Meyer, who continued her mouth-to-mouth breathing, with her son over eight miles of mountainous roads. An ambulance waited to take them on to Denver, twelve miles farther.

Fritz was on the hospital critical list for ten days—days that were spent in the hospital's Intensive Care Unit, where he received twenty-four-hour special care.

"I stayed right there with him in the hospital for the first three days," says Mrs. Meyer. "I just couldn't leave him all alone. He was so very sick those first few days and we were worried about the extent of his injuries. Severe internal concussions were the main trouble, and because of the danger of lung collapse, the little red-headed guy had not one bit of sedation for pain. He just had to tough it out. A tracheotomy tube, tubes in his lungs for draining, and a tube in his nose for intravenous feeding, plus the deep abrasions on his shoulders, head, and chest, really put him to the test. But the doctors said he never complained."

Thanks to Mrs. Meyer's presence of mind and the resuscitation which she did not abandon for even a moment on the long drive to the hospital, the doctors had a live, though very sick, child to treat. They used every facility the hospital had to offer to restore his health.

Three weeks later Fritz was back in school. The doctors who looked after him agreed that it was really his mother who had saved his life. Without the oxygen she provided by continuous mouth-to-mouth breathing, it would have been far too late to help Fritz by the time he arrived at the hospital.

The situation in which Elliott Spring, a forty-four-year-old houseware salesman in Miami, Florida, found himself on a hot August afternoon a couple of years ago, was not the kind that salesmen are expected to handle. Seated in the living room of

Louis Soto and his wife, Paula, Spring was giving a spiel on the virtues of his cookware. It looked like a sure sale. But suddenly Mrs. Soto, who had been admiring the merchandise, gave a sharp scream and ran from the room. She returned in a minute carrying a soaking wet baby who appeared to be dead. Intent on Spring's sales talk, she had completely forgotten that nine-month-old Christine was alone in the family bathtub.

Mr. Soto, galvanized into action, grabbed the baby and held her upside down in an attempt to expel some of the water she had swallowed, while Mrs. Soto stood crying hysterically. But fortunately Mr. Spring, who lives on a lake with his wife and two small sons, knew exactly what to do. Quickly taking the baby from the father and ordering him to call the police, he placed Christine on the floor and started mouth-to-mouth resuscitation. Because a baby's mouth is too small to allow much passage of air, Mr. Spring remembered to place his mouth tightly over the mouth and nose of the tiny child when he exhaled his breath. As he kept up the exhalation and inhalation at a steady pace, he was rewarded by seeing the infant's small chest rise and fall. Then the little hand began to move. Finally the baby gave a gasp.

But Christine was not in the clear, for she had swallowed a good deal of water. The police, who arrived within minutes, continued resuscitation as they raced to Jackson Memorial Hospital, where doctors provided intensive care. Thanks to Mr. Spring's presence of mind, doctors announced later that Christine's condition was improving and that she would recover.

Mr. Spring had learned resuscitation when he was in the Navy, but he credited his success in saving Christine's life to a film he had seen on TV that demonstrated the latest techniques of reversing death.

Drowning is one of the hazards that befall more than seven thousand men, women, and children each summer. However, the methods of resuscitating a person dragged from the water is far different and much more effective today than those commonly employed only a few years ago. Where rescuers used to concentrate mainly on trying to rid the body of excess water, the emphasis today is on getting oxygen into the lungs and restarting the heart as quickly as possible. People who drown die primarily of suffocation—water doesn't contain enough usable oxygen.

Experiments have demonstrated that in about half to three quarters of drowning cases neither the long-familiar Schaefer "prone-pressure" method nor the Holger Nielsen "back-pressure armlift method," as usually performed by trained rescuers, moved enough air into the lungs to sustain life. Mouth-to-mouth resuscitation, on the other hand, supplies up to twelve times the volume of air averaged by experts using the older methods.

Because the blood and tears of human beings have a salt content similar to that of ocean water, a drowning person has a better chance in salt water than in fresh water. For sea water tends to draw water out of the cells while fresh water readily permeates lung membranes, breaks down the red cells and often causes the heart to go into fibrillation (a useless twitching of the heart muscles). Drowning often calls for closed-heart massage as well as mouth-to-mouth breathing.

Because strangers did exactly the right thing at just the right times for her on a warm June afternoon, Betty Meulenberg, of Grand Rapids, Michigan, continued the merry, exciting business of being a twelve-year-old girl. Betty and three of her girl friends were swimming from the big float at Lamar Park Lake. They were in and out of the water so much that no one noticed when Betty didn't reappear on the raft. Fortunately, thirteen-year-old Gale Eckert, as at home in the water as a seal, was practicing skin diving. As he dove ten feet down he saw a strange object through his skin-diving mask. On closer investigation, he realized it was a small girl lying motionless at the bottom of the lake.

Eckert lost no time shooting to the surface to yell for help as loudly as he could. A lifeguard came splashing through the water within seconds. From the raft he spotted the outline of the body and quickly dove for it. Surfacing with the victim, he swam toward the shore and placed the girl on the sandy beach. She was blue; there was no pulse or respiration. Immediately the lifeguard started mouth-to-mouth resuscitation. But Betty didn't respond. An ambulance was on the way but, impeded by heavy traffic, it might be too late when it arrived.

Only a few feet away, Mrs. William Berry, a registered nurse, became aware of the commotion. She hurried to the spot and her trained eyes instantly recognized the gravity of the situation. Kneeling beside the lifeguard who was doing his best to revive Betty by forcing air into her lungs, the nurse started external heart massage—the second part of the resuscitative techniques recommended for drowning victims. Because the chest of the child was slight, the nurse, trained in modern first aid, used only one hand to compress the chest and force the blood to circulate.

In a few minutes a gasp escaped from the child. With her free hand, Mrs. Berry felt for a pulse. It was there, though feeble and faltering. Then, as she and the lifeguard continued their ministrations, the pulse grew stronger and the blueness began to recede from Betty's face.

Betty remained in a coma, and at the hospital she was immediately placed on an ice mattress to reduce her temperature and minimize the risk of neurological injury. Medication, oxygen, intravenous feedings were administered. Three days later Betty opened her eyes and smiled at her mother. After that, recovery was routine, thanks to the efficient preliminary assistance she had received.

Another child who owes his life to the fact that there was someone close by who knew how to apply resuscitation techniques is four-year-old Russell Dahlburg of New Jersey who fell into a brook near his home. At that precise moment, Mrs. Betty Thayer, herself a mother of three and a neighbor of the Dahlburgs, was finishing an article that explained the value of mouth-to-mouth resuscitation and how it should be applied.

Suddenly her four-year-old Jeffrey tore into the house

shouting about the boy in the brook. Mrs. Thayer ran to the stream. There was no sign of the child and she quickly dived in. She found Russell at the bottom of the brook which was five feet deep. But after she had pulled the child to safety she found, as she later stated, "I had a dead boy on my hands."

A physical therapist before her marriage, Mrs. Thayer now followed the directions of the article to the letter. Depositing the little boy on the ground, she placed one hand under his neck, thus tilting back his head and opening wide the airway which was clogged with mud and debris. Because it would be useless to try to force air into the lungs until the obstruction was removed, she took a clean handkerchief and carefully wiped away as much of the mud and water as she could reach. Not losing a minute, she then started mouth-to-mouth breathing. In-and-out, in-and-out, inhale-and-exhale, inhale-and-exhale—as she kept up the rhythm at twenty blows to the minute—she could see the child's chest move up and down and thus knew the air was getting through. (An adult needs only fifteen or sixteen blows a minute during mouth-to-mouth breathing but a child's respiration is faster and needs twenty.)

Neighbors had called the police but by the time they arrived, Russell was breathing again. Rushed to the hospital, he was put on the critical list because there was water in his lungs. Russell had a hard fight ahead of him, but the fact that he got immediate help when he was fished out of the pond turned the tide in his favor. He made a complete recovery.

Sometimes a few seconds of inattention is enough for catastrophe to befall a small child. On the morning of November 6, 1959, four-year-old Deborah Hodges was playing on the floor while her mother vacuumed the living room. Mrs. Hodges left the room for thirty seconds. When she came back little Deborah lay rigid and motionless on the floor. In the mother's brief absence, the child had touched both a wet mop and the vacuum cleaner, which was switched on.

Picking up her little girl, Mrs. Hodges ran out of the house and screamed for help. A neighbor raced the mother and child to a doctor's office, fortunately only a few blocks away. Mrs. Hodges later estimated that only three minutes elapsed between the accident and the time it took to reach the doctor's office.

Drs. Roy Halpern and R. O. A. Weber could find no heart-beat or respiration when they examined little Deborah. Her skin was blue and cold and the pupils of her eyes were dilated. She had all the symptoms of death. However, two weeks earlier the two doctors had viewed a film on resuscitation and had watched a similar case brought back to life. Quickly they decided to try the same techniques.

While one doctor inserted a tube through the mouth to establish a clear passage to the lungs, the other cut open the chest and started barehanded heart massage, which sent vital oxygen to the brain and kept the blood circulating. The next step was to restore the normal heartbeat. Luckily, the Riviera Hospital was across the street from the doctor's office.

Moments later, citizens of Torrance, California, witnessed a dramatic spectacle as the rescue team carried Deborah to the hospital. One doctor held the small girl in his arms while another blew air into her lungs through an intratracheal tube, and a third, with his hand in her open chest, massaged her heart. In the operating room her heart was defibrillated with an apparatus, and a normal heartbeat restored. Deborah, full of bounce and vitality, was discharged from the hospital eight days later.

Freak accidents are often the most dangerous. Being struck by lightning is a particularly terrifying experience. And it is usually fatal.

Ten-year-old Donald L. and several members of his scout troop were riding their bicycles on a secluded path in a Balti-more park on a hot July afternoon. By some fluke, Donald managed to get separated from the group. Suddenly a thunder-storm came up. Before he could take shelter, he was struck by lightning.

Ten minutes later—about 3:30 in the afternoon—a couple of

his scout friends found him. He lay, apparently dead, where he had fallen from his bike. The two boys bent over Donald, tried to get some response as they called his name and shook him. Suddenly recognizing the extreme seriousness of the situation, the boys recalled their training—when an accident causes death, resuscitation must be started immediately.

Kneeling at Donald's side, one of the boys placed his hand under his neck, thus tipping the head backwards and opening wide his mouth. He placed his other hand on the forehead and used his thumb to seal off the nose. He then took a deep breath, covered Donald's mouth tightly with his own and exhaled. Before taking his next breath he made sure that the air was moving Donald's chest. Encouraged, he continued his ministrations at a steady pace.

Meanwhile, his companion raced to the nearest telephone for help. He managed to reach Baltimore City Hospital and asked that an ambulance be sent immediately. The urgency in the boy's voice alerted the hospital. Unfortunately, when the ambulance arrived, it did not carry trained personnel to give proper resuscitation.

Undaunted, the boys accompanied their friends in the ambulance, continuing their ministrations. It was 3:45—twenty-five minutes after he was knocked unconscious by lightning—when Donald was carried into the emergency room. The boy looked beyond help. He was ashen gray, pulseless, flaccid and cold, his pupils widely dilated. A small burn on the left side of the scalp and on the left heel indicated the entrance and exit marks of the lightning current.

It looked hopeless but DOA—dead on arrival—is no longer accepted as final in many large hospitals until resuscitation is attempted. Pediatricians and anesthesiologists took over the job of trying to save Donald's life. To the doctors it was a fascinating case; there are few incidents in which a child who has been hit by lightning is brought to a hospital.

The doctors lost no time in starting resuscitation. A tracheotomy was immediately performed to allow a tube to be inserted into the airway through which the lungs could be kept oxygenated. At the same time, heart massage was started. It was almost an hour before Donald's heart began to beat feebly but it was an encouraging sign. To minimize the possibility of neurological damage Donald was placed on a mattress of crushed ice. Doctors find that even if brain injury has taken place, it can sometimes be counteracted by the use of hypothermia (near freezing.)

But Donald was still a long way from safety. He was placed in the Intensive Care Ward and the residents in pediatrics and anesthesiology spelled each other for the next seven days and nights while he remained unconscious and in critical condition. They made sure that he was never left alone for even a moment. Consultants in pediatrics and neurology supervised every detail of the therapy.

Donald received blood transfusions, infusions, miracle drugs. His response was limited but the doctors kept at it. Three days after the accident, Donald seemed to recognize his father. On the fifth day he mumbled an answer to a question put to him by a doctor. But for the most part he remained in a coma. His condition was further jeopardized when he developed bilateral pneumonia.

Hope that he would eventually recover became a certainty when he was able to whisper his age and correctly count the fingers on his hands. Donald became fully conscious on the tenth day, asked for food, and remained awake and rational from then on. He was still a very sick boy and had to be fed intravenously until the fifteenth day. More than three weeks passed before he was able to get out of bed. He was discharged from the hospital on the thirtieth day. An IQ test administered before he left showed the same result as one given at school three months prior to the accident.

The recovery, which was a complete success, was due, in part, to the devoted ministrations of his scout friends—they kept his body oxygenated during the crucial period immediately after the accident. Donald was back in his class when school started and has remained neurologically and mentally normal since that time.

Dr. Helen B. Taussig, professor emeritus of pediatrics at Johns Hopkins, writing in *Medical World News*, makes the point that few efforts are made to resuscitate persons who have been struck by lightning. Some recover spontaneously, but Dr. Taussig believes that many more could be saved if they received cardiac massage and prolonged artificial respiration.

It is particularly rewarding to salvage people who have been struck down by lightning because they usually suffer no impairment. In fact, according to Dr. Taussig: "If the 'dead' person revives, there is nothing in his appearance to indicate that anything unusual has happened to him. He travels on one of the few two-way streets to heaven. His trip may take days or weeks, but the chances are that he will be uninjured by the trip."

An extra factor played a role in the successful resuscitation of the youngsters involved in the following cases. Each of the children drowned during bitter cold weather; each was dead for more than twenty-five minutes. In each case hypothermia—near freezing—played a significant role in preserving their lives. Not only were the children's lives saved but hypothermia prevented neurological damage.

In March, 1962, with a bitter wind blowing and the temperature below zero, five-year-old Roger Arntsen of Trondheim, Norway, fell into the ice-choked Nidelven River. It was twenty-two minutes before he was pulled out from beneath the ice. The policeman who rescued him attempted mouth-to-mouth breathing while in the river, but was not successful because the boy's mouth and windpipe were clogged with vomitus.

When Dr. Tone Dahl Kvittingen arrived ten minutes later the boy had been clinically dead for thirty-two minutes. His skin was blue, his eyes widely dilated and there was absolutely no pulse. Though his condition seemed hopeless, Roger had one factor going for him. The raw March wind, which was a frigid 14° Fahrenheit, and the river at close to 32°, were in the little boy's favor. When he lost his hold on the ice and fell in, he was already exhausted and chilled; doctors later reasoned that he probably did not fight much for air, and as a result inhaled less water than he might have.

The icy river soon dropped his body temperature below 75°, so that when he drowned and circulation stopped, his brain suffered less from oxygen deprivation than it would have at normal body heat. But this was about the only optimistic item that the doctors working over him could find.

In spite of the time elapsed since the boy had plunged into the water, Dr. Kvittingen started immediate resuscitation. He turned Roger upside down to get rid of as much water as possible, then started artificial respiration with a tube down the boy's windpipe. On the way to the hospital the doctor maintained closed heart massage, thus forcing blood in and out of the heart.

At Central Hospital the method of resuscitation became more complicated and intense. A special electrode needle, pushed right through the chest wall into the heart, failed to detect any beat. Nevertheless, doctors, spelling each other, continued externally massaging the heart without letup. They cut a hole in Roger's neck to pass a tube down his windpipe, through which they extracted more vomit. Roger also received a blood transfusion. But two and a half hours went by before his heart resumed a natural beat. Soon after that he began to breathe for himself.

But his condition remained critical. Roger ran a high temperature, went into shock, suffered seizures and severe episodes of pulmonary edema. His kidneys failed and he could not swallow food. Roger received a whole pharmacopeia of drugs as well as intensive care from the medical staff.

A week later, when the air tube was taken out and Roger could be fed by mouth, he seemed on the mend. But his travail had not ended. Eleven days after the drowning the boy suddenly entered a crisis. The doctors still cannot pinpoint the cause of his relapse, but Roger lost consciouness and began to shriek incoherently. He thrashed around so violently that for two weeks he had to be constantly sedated.

For a month it seemed that Roger's brain had been all but destroyed. He developed an enormous appetite and opened his mouth for food whenever his lips were touched. He went blind, and fell on his face against the bedpost when he sat up.

Then, six weeks after his accident, Roger's mental condition improved as inexplicably as it had deteriorated. He began to speak. Soon after that he regained vision for near objects, and later for distant ones. He seemed to be normal in every way.

Roger was discharged ten weeks after the drowning. Retested six months later, doctors found his neurological status, including vision, was completely normal.

Doctors reasoned that the cooling of the child's body while under the ice—and the hypothermia that was used during treatment—played an important role in the successful outcome.

"We are learning that there are no set rules," said Dr. Kvittingen.

In Hamburg, Germany, a five-year-old boy trying to cross the Alster River which was frozen over disappeared under the thick icy covering. Other children playing nearby called to passersby for aid. Several people responded, but were unable to find a trace of the child.

It was more than twenty minutes before the fire brigade personnel who had been summoned found him. The temperature was a frigid 8°. The child was considered dead and no revival measures were attempted during the trip to Eppendorf Hospital. The medical staff, however, started immediate resuscitation. They estimated that the child had been in clinical death for more than a half hour.

The water was quickly sucked out of the boy's trachea, a tube placed down his windpipe, his soaked clothing removed and heart massage started. Oxygen was continually fed into the windpipe and intracardiac injections of adrenaline were administered—all without the slightest effect.

After fifty minutes and another intracardiac injection of adrenaline, ventricular fibrillation set in for about ten minutes. After that there were no signs of life.

It looked hopeless to all the doctors assembled around the boy—except a woman physician who was pregnant. She could not bear to declare the child dead. Hour after hour she continued massaging the heart. To help her along, numerous injections of procaine, a heart rhythm regulator, calcium gluconate, and sodium bicarbonate, to buffer the acid condition that accompanies clinical death, were given to the boy.

Four hours later a weak and fluttery heartbeat was finally restored. Intracardiac injection of stimulating drugs were again used, but the boy's condition did not improve. As a last resort, an internal pacemaker was inserted. Forty-five minutes later it was turned off when the boy's heart rate and blood pressure became normal.

But the child was still very ill. He ran a high temperature and his voice was very hoarse. Pink frothy secretion was evident at the mouth and nose and examination showed that the lungs had been damaged by the fresh water of the icy river. Chest X rays revealed pulmonary edema (congestion of the lungs).

Finally, seventeen hours after he had regained consciousness the boy was neurologically normal, could give rational answers, and was able to take nourishment. He remained in the hospital for eight weeks. Upon discharge his only residual difficulty was slight paralysis of the small muscles of one hand. His intelligence and behavior were completely normal. Testing of his IQ showed it to be the same as before the accident.

The doctors who worked with the child emphasize that the revival period at normal temperature can be measured in minutes; the icy temperature undoubtedly made possible the complete recovery of the boy even after more than five hours of clinical death.

In sharp contrast was the case of six-year-old Bonnie Lundgren, who wandered away from a ski lodge in New Hampshire. Bonnie was looking for her parents on the ski slopes, but they had long since returned to the lodge and were having a drink in the lounge. They, in turn, thought their small daughter was being cared for by one of the maids.

Bonnie soon became lost. As she trudged on and on, daylight faded and it began to snow. When Bonnie was missed six hundred volunteers turned out to scour the countryside. The snow was heavy and the searchers had difficulty finding any leads. It was early morning when Bonnie was found under a snowbank. She was literally frozen stiff.

The local doctor looked with dismay at the small frozen body.

"It's not a doctor she needs," he muttered, as he methodically checked her pulse and respiration and found both nonexistent. He had no training in modern resuscitation. Instead, he tried an injection of adrenalin to start the heart. When it failed to work, he declared the child dead.

It was doubly heartbreaking for the parents when their doctor in New York told them: "But she could have been saved. If she had received proper resuscitation, she could probably have been brought back to life. And she would have been perfectly all right for the severe cold would have protected her from brain injury."

5.

HEART FAILURE: AMERICA'S NUMBER ONE KILLER

Among those who stood up to cheer the boys of the visiting basketball team—many of whom he had known since childhood and had watched develop scholastically and athletically—was Wayne Rulon, vice-principal of Brookfield High School. Suddenly his cheer turned to a moan. His hands clutched at his chest. Hemmed in by students, he knew he had to have air. Unsteadily he made for the aisle. As he stumbled forward unbearable pain blotted out the noise and the crowd. He fell heavily to the floor.

It appeared to be an accident. But to Philip Couch, seated nearby, it looked ominous. As he bent over Rulon, he could discern no heartbeat, no sign of respiration. In the heat of the game the vice-principal had met sudden death.

Couch was quickly joined by explorer scout Richy Moore, school nurse Maudie Ross, and the Reverend Tom Turner of Linneus. Carefully they lifted the stricken man and carried him out of the noisy gymnasium into an adjoining alcove.

Trained as a scout master, Couch had some knowledge of first aid. But as he looked down at Rulon he realized that the type of first aid he had been taught was not good enough. What was needed was the new type of resuscitation that only recently had been introduced at the Johns Hopkins Medical Center and approved by the American Heart and the American Medical associations. Only a few days earlier he had read an article which carefully described how closed-heart massage was performed. The article stated that if applied quickly enough it could restore life to a person in clinical death.

Couch knew that this type of resuscitation, though it can be performed by laymen, usually requires practice. Closed-heart massage, if not properly executed could—he knew—cause breakage of ribs or damage the liver or other organs.

But he had to try. Far better for his friend to land in the hospital with a broken rib than in the morgue with his ribs intact. His years of training were in his favor. As he had read the article, his mind's eye had carefully visualized each step. Now his hands instinctively followed through.

Kneeling at the side of the striken man so that he could use his entire weight in applying pressure, he placed the heel of his left hand on the lower end of the breastbone. He made sure that his fingers were opened and raised so that he would not depress the ribs.

He then placed the heel of his right hand on top of the left and pressed down with all his strength. After each stroke he lifted both hands slightly to allow the chest to expand. This pressure forced blood to circulate from the heart to the brain; removing pressure allowed the heart to refill. He repeated this procedure at the rate of once a second.

As Couch worked steadily and firmly, explorer scout Moore tilted back the head of the stricken man and started mouth-to-mouth breathing. Rulon was getting oxygen to his lungs and blood to his brain, the two elements that would keep him alive until trained medical men could take over.

By the time an ambulance arrived Mr. Rulon was breathing and his heart was beating faintly. Taken to Pershing Memorial Hospital, Rulon received the definitive medical care that is so important after a heart attack. He remained a patient in the hospital for several weeks. Thanks to the quick thinking of his friends he made an excellent recovery.

On a bright March afternoon in 1964 during baseball spring

training in Tucson, Arizona, Birdie Tebbetts, manager of the Cleveland Indians, felt tired as he returned to his motel room. It had been a full day. Getting the team in shape was always a period of tension.

There was no warning, no foretelling symptom. The pain struck his chest with stunning intensity. As he fell to the floor his senses were acute and sharp. He recognized the onset of a full-scale heart attack.

The deep, penetrating pain made every breath a torture. But his mind, working rapidly, told him he had to get help—had to leave one last message for his family.

Regis McAuley, sports editor of the Cleveland *Plain Dealer* heard his cry and rushed to his aid. The crushing pain made speech a burden Tebbetts could hardly bear. Holding on to consciousness with every ounce of will power, Tebbetts gasped: "This is it. . . . My brother died of a heart attack. . . . Bring my kids here; it'll be the last time. . . ."

Tebbetts was not exaggerating. He was, indeed, in dire trouble. He lost consciousness and it looked like the end. The oldest of human emotions were exposed—a man struck down in his prime, a wife alone, children wondering if they would ever see their father again.

But fortunately McAuley knew the procedure of the new revival tactics. He lost no time. For forty-five minutes McAuley worked on Tebbetts, first giving three strong blows to his lungs, then shifting to the chest and doing fifteen strong heart compressions. The pressure on Tebbetts' chest forced an artificial heartbeat, expelled blood out of the heart into the arteries; the mouth-to-mouth resuscitation aerated the lungs. The blue color had begun to recede and the heart to come back when a doctor took over.

Four months later Tebbetts was back on the ball field with the Indians!

All-American football player, Lee Grosscup, famed for his daring plays on the gridiron made the most dramatic headline of his career not as quarterback at the University of Utah, but when he used his knowledge of resuscitation to save the life of his father.

Clyde Grosscup and his wife, of Santa Monica, California, were visiting their famous son in Salt Lake City where he was finishing his studies at the university. Accompanied by his wife and his parents, Lee was driving along the foot of the Wasatch Mountains when the older man suddenly collapsed. Without losing a moment the young football star propped his father's legs up on a car seat and began applying resuscitation.

Deputy Sheriff Bob Jack, who was eventually flagged down by one of the other passengers in the car, said, "Lee's quick action in applying mouth-to-mouth breathing saved his father's life. When I got there, you could hardly find a pulse." Mr. Grosscup recuperated at Latter-Day Saints Hospital.

Of all the debilitating and degenerative diseases, heart failure is the greatest killer. It is estimated that twenty million Americans suffer from heart trouble. During the coming year some 700,000 of these—many of them unaware that there is anything wrong with their hearts—will die of coronary heart disease and sudden cardiac arrest. Yet most cardiologists today agree that more than *50 percent of the men and women who die suddenly of heart attack could be saved and given years of life if resuscitation was promptly instituted.*

Recent studies have shown that sudden death can occur from minimal myocardial damage. Provided with a second chance, these hearts can beat again for many years. Pointing up the needless waste of sudden death from heart failure is a study by Dr. Lester Adelson, Medical Examiner of Cleveland. Dr. Adelson performed five hundred autopsies on heart victims—all of them men who died during their every-day activities, in their offices, in public buildings, in their homes.

The findings showed that 63 percent of these men could have been revived had they received help in time. The pathological findings showed no gross heart damage in these victims, nor was there any evidence of heart failure. The report stated: "Under proper conditions, these deaths could have been reversed and their lives saved."

"Knowledge of the heart has now reached a point where it can be restarted almost at will," says Dr. Claude S. Beck, Chief of Cardiac Surgery at Western Reserve University in Cleveland, Ohio. Dr. Beck compares the heart to a clock which sometimes needs only a little push to start it ticking again. But the push must be given quickly or it will be too late.

The safest place to die is in the operating room. There trained personnel know how to cope with a crisis; surgeon, anesthetists, and nurses are all prepared to fight for life.

Of the thousands of people who have been brought back from sudden death and have continued to live normally, the vast majority owe their added years to the brilliant life-saving techniques that have come into use during the last two decades.

In 1947, the first time a patient who died on the operating table was brought back by a surgeon's ingenuity, medical history was made. The patient was fourteen-year-old Richard Heyard, undergoing an operation at Western University Hospital to repair a very serious malformation of the chest. The surgeon was Dr. Beck, who had put in an active lifetime of research on the heart. Richard Heyard was doing fine—or so it seemed to the surgical team—when suddenly his heart began fibrillating, a situation which in those days usually meant the patient was irrevocably dead.

But this time Dr. Beck, who had fought sudden death on the operating table since his early days as a student, was prepared. For months he had worked on a homemade shocking device, or defibrillator, with a pair of electrodes shaped like round spatulas. Again and again he had experimented on animals. Now as he looked down at the boy dead on the table, he decided the time had come to put it to use on a human being. Placing the electrodes on either side of the heart, he switched on the current for a brief second. The boy's heart was shocked to a standstill.

A few minutes later the heart was once more convulsing wildly. Electric shock was again applied. For the next seventy-five minutes, Dr. Beck massaged the heart until it returned to a coordinated beat. He then finished the operation.

In spite of his near-death on the operating table, young Heyard had an uneventful recovery. He left the hospital a month later and that fall entered the seventh grade. Subsequently, he played three and one-half years of varsity basketball, in high school. Today he is a draftsman in Canton, Ohio, healthy, married, and the father of a son.

The first resuscitation of heart failure *outside* an operating room occurred eight years later. On the morning of June 21, 1955, Dr. Albert T. Ransone had an electrocardiogram at Cleveland's Western Reserve University Hospital. Fully dressed, he was just leaving the building when he keeled over with a coronary attack. Dr. Ransone's death would have been complete within minutes if he had walked the few more steps that would have taken him outside the hospital building. But falling as he did in the doorway, he was surrounded by doctors almost immediately.

Dr. Eldon C. Weckesser, who ran to his side, found no pulse or respiration. There was no time to take him to the operating room, to arrange for sterilization, for the meticulous techniques that are routine there. With the help of other doctors, he had Dr. Ransone moved to a side corridor, where he was placed on the bare floor. In two minutes, Dr. Weckesser had slashed open the chest with the first instrument he could lay his hands on while another doctor established an airway and started pumping oxygen into the stricken man's lungs.

With the chest opened, it was obvious that Dr. Ransone had been slugged by a massive heart attack. Dr. Weckesser started massaging the heart but it began to fibrillate. The convulsions were getting stronger in spite of the massage and would undoubtedly have ended in biological death very quickly, for the fibrillating heart rarely responds to heart massage alone. Even strong drugs given by injections which reduce the myocardial irritability often fail.

Fortunately Dr. Beck was in the building. Using an electric defibrillator—the same one he had used for the first time on young Heyard—he brought the jiggling heart out of its tailspin. Routine in most hospitals today, the use of the defibrillator was considered a dramatically daring procedure in 1955. But it worked. The heart stopped fibrillating and came to a standstill and Dr. Beck massaged it back to its normal rhythm.

As a result of the resuscitation that was so daringly applied, Dr. Ransone landed in the recovery ward instead of the morgue. He was back at his medical practice six weeks later. In 1964, at seventy-one, Dr. Ransone moved to an active, happy retirement in Florida where he remains in excellent health.

One of the few persons who passed into clinical death outside a hospital and lived to tell about it was Mr. Nicholas Muray, well-known photographer and socialite. In a dramatic episode that makes the heroic efforts of Dr. Casey and Dr. Kildare pale by comparison, Mr. Muray had his death reversed by a young doctor who had just finished his residency at the Bronx Veterans Hospital.

At six-thirty on the evening of February 6, 1961, Mr. Muray, then sixty-nine, had just finished an hour's fencing at the New York Athletic Club. Although he had a history of heart trouble—he had suffered a heart attack three years earlier—Mr. Muray had recovered sufficiently to lead an active life. He was pleasantly tired as he walked away from the arena. Suddenly he staggered and fell to the floor. Dr. Barry Pariser, doing calisthenics nearby, ran to his side. The stricken man had no pulse, no respiration. Death had come to Mr. Muray without warning.

Dr. Pariser, who specialized in diseases of the eye, ear, nose, and throat, had received training in resuscitative techniques. Only a few weeks before he had massaged back to life the heart of a six-year-old child who had died on the operating table. But all of Dr. Pariser's experience had been in the operating theater where every possible type of equipment was instantly available, where a seasoned staff of surgeons was present to give advice and help.

Nevertheless, as Dr. Pariser looked down at Mr. Muray, he knew that the stricken man's only chance lay in immediate resuscitation before the vital tissues of the brain died. He quickly began mouth-to-mouth breathing, alternating with closed-chest massage. When this did not suffice, another man took over the mouth-to-mouth breathing. Dr. Pariser borrowed a pocket knife from one of the members who clustered about, slashed open the chest and with his bare hands began rhymically to squeeze the heart.

Though a call for an ambulance had gone out almost as soon as Mr. Muray collapsed, it was forty-five minutes before it arrived. New York City, which has a central pooling system for ambulances, allots them as the calls come in. On the night of Mr. Muray's brush with death, all the ambulances were busy with calls from hospitals on the other side of the city. Had he received no help while he waited, Mr. Muray's first stop would undoubtedly have been the morgue—the fate of so many victims of sudden death.

When the ambulance did arrive, Mr. Muray was carefully lifted by the attendants while Dr. Pariser continued to manipulate the heart. On the way to the hospital, the victim's heart began to beat faintly and the blue that tinged his face slowly receded. He was not out of danger, however. But Dr. Pariser and his assistant had bought vital time—time in which his brain was kept alive, thus making it possible for specialists to take over the job.

Dr. Pariser continued to massage Mr. Muray's heart as he was lifted out of the ambulance and carried into the elevator that took him to the operating room of the hospital. A team of surgeons and doctors headed by Mr. Muray's own cardiologist and internist, Dr. Walter Wichern and Dr. Frank F. Iaquinta, had everything set up. The surgical staff was scrubbed and ready, the operating room in perfect order.

Mr. Muray still had a long way to go. As the doctors worked over him, his heart went into fibrillation. He suffered attacks of ventricular tachycardia in which his heart raced wildly and he developed hypotension—extremely low blood pressure. Drugs, electric shock, intravenous fluids—all were used. After eleven failures, the normal rhythm of his heart was finally established.

The persistent efforts of the medical staff paid off. The heart was stabilized, the wound closed and Mr. Muray was moved to the Intensive Care Unit. Though he remained in the hospital five weeks, he was fully alert the day after his sudden collapse. When he left the hospital, his heart was in better condition than it had been for some time. The cardiogram showed the heart had completely healed.

A clean bill of health by a doctor does not, in our present state of medical knowledge, guarantee that a heart attack will not strike at any moment.

Fifty-five-year-old William L. Rieth, a sales manager of Cleveland, Ohio, and his wife were planning their first trip to Europe the summer of 1959. Life looked good as they studied travel folders, made reservations, and prepared for a tour that would take them to several countries. Two weeks before they were scheduled to sail, the couple received the necessary immunization shots. Mr. Rieth decided that he might as well have a complete overhauling as he had not undergone a physical checkup in some time. The results of all tests were uniformly excellent. Rieth was apparently in splendid health. But a few days before they were ready to leave for Europe, Mr. Rieth began to feel ill.

"I thought it might be a reaction to the shots," Mr. Rieth recalled. He stopped in to see his doctor. After listening to Mr. Rieth's symptoms, the doctor gave him an examination. Rieth had suffered a heart attack!

"I want you to go to the hospital immediately," the doctor told him.

Rieth telephoned his wife, gave her the news and asked her to meet him at Western Reserve Hospital, where a bed was waiting for him.

Silent coronary artery disease is present in a very large percentage of the population, according to a survey recently conducted by Drs. Arthur M. Master and Arthur J. Geller of New York. In their report the doctors stated that many persons with severe arteriosclerosis and with myocardial infarction never experience a chest pain.

Nor can one count on the electrocardiogram or other diagnostic tools to bring the trouble to light. The doctors indicated, for instance, that the EKG is negative in 50 to 80 percent of proved cases of angina pectoris. New machines and methods may some day make it possible to foretell with certainty when a heart attack will strike, but as of now, the best method of fighting fatal attacks is to give a second chance to the heart that still has mileage in it.

Rieth was frightened by the words "heart attack" but after he'd been in bed three days, he felt so rested he decided it couldn't have been too serious. When his tray came around, he did full justice to the fish dinner. It was only minutes later that his roommate noticed that Rieth had "gone out." He rang for a nurse and yelled at the same time. A nurse came running in. Bending over the prone form, she found no pulse or respiration and immediately started mouth-to-mouth breathing.

Meanwhile, another nurse, who had heard the commotion, had put the alert on the intercom. Within minutes doctors and nurses from all over the hospital had converged at the bedside of Mr. Rieth. A doctor quickly opened the chest and started massaging the heart. The heart team that responded to the call connected the electrocardiograph which acts as a monitor during resuscitation. The heart was fibrillating. Dr. Claude Beck, who was on the scene, used a defibrillator while other doctors managed the oxygen supply, cut down a vein for intravenous feeding, set up a supply of necessary drugs.

Close to forty minutes transpired before Rieth recovered

consciousness. He seemed confused and drowsy. Mrs. Rieth was terrified. Had his brain been adversely affected by the long period of unconsciousness? The next morning her husband looked brighter. She decided to find out for herself whether there had been any brain damage.

"Bill, what's the definition of ecology?" she asked casually.

Mr. Rieth did not seem to think that a strange question. "Ecology," he explained, "is the relation of environment to the organism." Mrs. Rieth breathed a sigh of relief. It was obvious there was nothing wrong with his brain.

Mr. Rieth left the hospital at the end of six weeks. He has been in excellent health since.

The symptoms that presage a heart attack vary greatly—ranging from a pain in the left arm to what most people diagnose as a bad attack of indigestion. This was what Mr. M., a forty-year-old mail carrier, thought he was troubled with on the morning of May 15, 1962, when he began experiencing abdominal pain. He kept thinking that if he could get to a drugstore and take some simple medication he would feel better, but he was in the middle of his route and there wasn't a drugstore in sight. In addition to the pain, he felt nauseous and faint.

As he stopped to deliver the mail at the office of Drs. Asher and Martin M. Black, he mentioned to the nurse that he felt dizzy and sick. Noting his extreme pallor, the nurse immediately notified the doctors who ushered him into an examining room. But Mr. M. had barely been placed on an examining table when he lost consciousness and stopped breathing. His pupils dilated widely and the doctors could detect no heart sounds or pulse rate.

While one doctor immediately started mouth-to-mouth breathing, the other began external cardiac massage. Meanwhile, a nurse quickly prepared an injection of epinephrine which was administered intravenously. Within a minute after the injection, the doctors noted that the pupils were no longer dilated. Encouraged, they continued with mouth-to-mouth respiration and external cardiac massage for thirty minutes when an ambulance arrived. They kept up their first-aid techniques en route to the hospital where a trained team waited to take over.

At the hospital, tracheal intubation was performed at the same time that massage was maintained. An electrocardiogram revealed ventricular fibrillation so electric defibrillation was undertaken. But the heart, which was suffering from an acute myocardial infarction, did not respond well. In all, five electric shocks were given and a number of medications injected intravenously. Blood pressure, which was previously unobtainable, rose to 70 over 56. At this point, the patient was able to breathe for himself. A few minutes later, after a generalized convulsion which lasted for fifty seconds, he became conscious and recognized his attending physician. He had been unconscious for fifty-five minutes.

In the Intensive Care Unit, Mr. M. remained conscious and cooperative. But at 7 P.M.—four and a half hours after he first met clinical death—the electrocardiogram, which acts as a monitor to a severely sick heart, again showed ventricular fibrillation. Within a minute, Mr. M. went into cardiac arrest—the second death within a few hours. Once more mouth-to-mouth respiration and external cardiac massage was instituted and electric defibrillation undertaken. Thirty minutes later, Mr. M. again returned to life.

During his stay in the hospital for the next six weeks, Mr. M. had many set-backs, including hypotension, an attack of tachycardia (rapid heartbeat), and a harsh friction rub in the chest. But by May 24, nine days after entering the hospital, most of his troubles began to disappear and the electrocardiogram showed a regular rhythm.

Mr. M. was discharged from the hospital on June 10. Today he is back on his mail-carrying route, which includes the office of the Drs. Black.

Mr. M. had luck on his side when trouble struck. Not only was he able to reach a doctor at the crucial time, but the physicians who took charge of him were trained in the art of resuscitation. Experts in the field are campaigning for more intensive training in resuscitative techniques of doctors throughout the country. Such a universal program will save more lives, they believe, than the most effective miracle drug ever produced.

Why does one person who seemingly has little chance of survival make a comeback while another whose condition is not as serious, succumbs quickly though both received medical care? The answer to that question is not yet known, for doctors are aware that there are many things going on in the heart that do not show up on the electrocardiogram. Nor is it visible to the human eye. But all too often, when victory is snatched from the hands of death, it becomes very clear that the devoted and untiring efforts of the physician played a major part in the outcome.

When Charles Welsh, a dentist of Cheyenne, Wyoming, suddenly became ill he immediately called Dr. Ben M. Leeper, a well-known internist and heart specialist. In less than ten minutes Leeper reached the apartment where Welsh, a fifty-nine-year-old bachelor, lived alone. A quick examination showed that Dr. Welsh had suffered a mild heart attack—his heart was racing wildly with ventricular tachycardia, an abnormally fast heartbeat. Dr. Leeper called an ambulance and had Welsh installed at De Paul Hospital.

Upon reexamination Dr. Leeper found that a small clot had blocked off the flow of blood to a portion of Welch's heart muscle, causing a small part of it to die. This in itself is not too serious but in Welsh's case the dying muscle began to issue rapid electrical impulses that took control of the heart away from the pacemaker which ordinarily controls the electrical impulse of the heart.

Dr. Leeper ordered oxygen and put the patient on intravenous quinidine, a drug which would quiet the heart. But Welsh's heart didn't respond too well. When a priest came to the room Dr. Welsh received absolution. Fifteen minutes later Welsh suddenly stopped breathing and his heart stopped beating. It was

the first of a series of death episodes. Instantly Dr. Leeper went
into action. There was no time to call a surgeon or worry about
the niceties of sterilization. Grabbing a pair of scissors he cut a
ten-inch incision in the patient's chest. Reaching into the chest
cavity with his bare hands he began squeezing the heart at the
rate of once a second. At the same time a floor nurse who had
responded to his call was doing mouth-to-mouth resuscitation.
Within a few minutes Welsh started normal, involuntary breathing and regained consciousness. Dr. John Gramlich responded
in answer to Dr. Leeper's call for a surgeon to suture the patient's
chest, but advised against subjecting the patient to the shock of
anesthesia. He closed the wound with adhesive tape. This decision probably saved Welsh's life. Only a few minutes after the
chest was taped Welsh once more lapsed into unconsciousness
and suffered a second cardiac arrest.

Ripping off the adhesive tape Dr. Gramlich began massaging
the heart while Dr. Leeper blew air into the patient's lungs. After
about fifteen minutes, Welsh revived. Coming out of an excruciating ordeal he was exhausted and frightened, but Dr. Leeper
assured him he was doing fine. But the physician did not feel as
sanguine as he sounded. He had never known a patient who had
managed to survive more than two heart arrests.

Welsh's condition seemed improved but Dr. Leeper took no
chances. He increased the dose of quinidine and through the
long night he kept vigil, carefully checking the EKG tape, which
is usually done for at least twenty-five hours after a heart has
been restarted. Occasionally he used a cardioscope, a machine
that registers heart activity in the form of a dancing line of light
on a radarlike screen. The patient seemed to be responding to
the medication. The rhythm of his heart continued normal.

But this proved to be only an interval. At noon the next
day Charles Welsh suddenly went out again. Dr. Walter Long
was in the room at the time—he had stopped by to see how the
patient was making out—and took over the job of providing
oxygen while Dr. Leeper manipulated the heart to restart cir-

culation. But the rhythm of the heart didn't return for the heart had gone into fibrillation.

Dr. Leeper, still massaging the heart, asked the nurse to prepare the electric defibrillator in order to shock the heart back into rhythmic action. Placing two spoonlike electrodes of the machine against Welsh's heart, Dr. Leeper and Dr. Long quickly stepped back for a few seconds to avoid being shocked themselves. The current was turned on for a tenth of a second. But the heart continued its wild oscillation. The charge was increased to 140 volts. The heart paused, then started quivering again. Six electric jolts had to be given in quick succession before the heart stabilized. Dr. Leeper resumed massaging the heart which now began to beat rhythmically. Charles Welsh opened his eyes. But his ordeal was still not over. Twice more within the hour Welsh went into fibrillation and with the aid of the electric defibrillator came back again.

A colleague urged Dr. Leeper to give up, stating that he was dealing with a fatal condition and was only putting the patient through unnecessary suffering.

Welsh himself had come to the same conclusion. After the fifth attack he opened his eyes and pleaded with Leeper to let him go. "It's not worth it, Doc. Quit trying," he told Leeper.

But Dr. Leeper had a stubborn streak that refused to admit failure. He recognized that Welsh's condition was worsening. But as long as there was even the slimmest chance, he couldn't give up.

Charlie Welsh had been in deep trouble since he entered the hospital. But at 7:40 P.M. of the second day the seventh and worst episode occurred. There was a seeming finality to the unequal battle when Charlie suddenly went into the classic death throes. As the last breath rattled in his throat he vomited blood and turned blue. Dr. Leeper tore off the chest tape and slid his hand around the heart. This sort of erratic stopping and starting is a big strain on the heart. With each stoppage, the odds against restarting mount. As Dr. Leeper massaged the heart it felt like quivering gelatin in his palm. As he kept gently squeezing Dr. Leeper prayed for help. And when Charlie suddenly breathed and opened his eyes, Dr. Leeper silently thanked God. But Welsh was tired to death. "Doc, let me die," he pleaded.

But Dr. Leeper had fought too long and too hard to give up now. "You'll be all right," he assured his patient, and went right on planning for each emergency as it presented itself. The problems were staggering. The weakened heart could not afford another bout of fibrillation. Dr. Leeper switched from quinidine to procaine amide, which has proven more successful in preventing fibrillation. But procaine amide like many strong medications has the ability to kill as well as heal. Unless he could balance the need exactly a toxic reaction could prove fatal.

Dr. Leeper began with a double dose of 200 mgs. and for a few minutes the heart beat regularly. But as the minutes passed the heartbeat on the screen of the cardioscope began to skip around, which meant another episode of fibrillation was coming. Dr. Leeper quickly stepped up the dosage to 400 mgs. then 500, 600, and 700. For five minutes the heart would beat regularly, then grow erratic. Fearful but determined he increased the dose to 800. At any moment, if Welsh didn't die of a fibrillating heart, he could succumb from an overdose of procaine amide. But Dr. Leeper felt he had no other recourse but to keep on with the medication. By 1 A.M. he was pouring 1,150 mgs. of procaine amide an hour into the patient. Like a man on a tight rope Leeper kept balancing the medication against the onslaught of fibrillation. Either another attack of fibrillation or an overdose of the medication could result in instant death.

During the long night Welsh's heart began missing beats. It looked as if the drug had so dulled the reflexes of the heart that it would simply stop. But the beat came back. Dr. Leeper kept struggling to keep the heart's action and the drug in balance, increasing the dosage when the heartbeat grew rapid, cutting it when the beat faltered.

And then it was as if a miracle had happened. After two long days and three full nights Charlie's heart began to rally.

The beat became stronger and the rhythm smoother. Leeper, who had not had even a moment's rest since he brought Charlie Welsh into the hospital, felt encouraged enough to get some sleep on a cot in the corridor outside his patient's room. His nurse was told to wake him every hour. Welsh continued to make progress and the following night Welsh had the nurse wake him every two hours.

Two days later Welsh's heart was strong enough to withstand the suturing of his chest. Welsh continued to thrive and Leeper felt it safe to visit his home for a few hours. But he returned that evening and continued his vigil. It was eight days—days in which Dr. Leeper spent almost every waking hour fighting to keep Charlie Welsh alive—before Dr. Leeper felt it safe to resume his normal schedule. The patient's life was saved.

Forty-six days after the original bout Welsh walked out of the hospital. His doctor was well satisfied and assured his patient that he had little to worry about. His heart had mended well and he could look forward to years of health.

Charlie Welsh, given a second chance at life, is finding it wonderful. Everything has taken on a new value—the handshake of a friend, the sound of voices, the feel of sunshine on his face. And when Welsh talks of his hospital stay and his long travail it is Dr. Leeper that he credits with the victory.

"That darn Ben Leeper—he wouldn't quit," he says. "And he wouldn't let me quit."

Equally amazing is the medical history of Delroy Outhouse of Dartmouth, Nova Scotia, who suffered from three severe heart conditions, at times concurrently and each potentially fatal. During his fight for survival, Mr. Outhouse died eleven times!

A forty-six-year-old Canadian, Mr. Outhouse, was admitted to Victoria General Hospital in Halifax with what was first diagnosed as aortic stenosia—a narrowing of the valve opening between the lower left chamber of the heart and the large artery called the aorta. Arrangements were made to transfer him to

Toronto General Hospital for insertion of a prosthetic aortic valve.

Before he could be transferred, however, Mr. Outhouse suffered a complete heart block and arrest. It proved to be the first of many deaths. Had it occurred a few years earlier, it might well have been the end of the story. But resuscitation techniques are practiced routinely at Victoria General. In less than a minute help had arrived. Under the direction of Dr. Paul Landrigan, the heartbeat was restored with closed-chest massage. But the surgeon, realizing that Outhouse would not survive the journey to Toronto without further help, set about implanting an internal pacemaker electrode. During the five-hour procedure, the patient's heart stopped nine times—each time resuscitation techniques, which ranged from oxygen and heart massage to electric shock and drugs, were effectively applied.

Mr. Outhouse, who was conscious during most of the time, remembers that each death episode was preceded by a "queer burning feeling that would pass down my back and I'd know I was going out." At other intervals he felt warm and dizzy. While on the operating table, he saw a doctor shaking his head at another doctor in a melancholy way and knew they didn't expect him to last long. But like most people in critical condition, he felt aloof from the situation—as if the doctors were referring to someone else.

"It didn't bother me any," he later explained. "I knew I was going out and everything would go black."

But Mr. Outhouse, much to his and the doctors' surprise, always managed to come back. Finally the external transistorized pacemaker was attached to the electrode in his heart and he was ready to be flown to Toronto. But no commercial airline would take the risk of flying a man who might suffer a heart attack that would prove fatal. The Royal Canadian Air Force, therefore, finally flew him on a mission of mercy.

At the Toronto hospital where Mr. Outhouse was to be operated on by Dr. Douglas Wigle, his heart suddenly resumed a normal rhythm. An electrocardiogram revealed he had suffered a myocardial infarction—death of an area of the heart muscle—in addition to the heart block. This meant that the operation had to be put off for six weeks while the muscle healed. But Mr. Outhouse hadn't yet run the full gamut of bad luck. While in bed his movements dislodged the electrode in the ventricle, and his heart promptly stopped. This time he was clinically dead for two and a half minutes before resuscitation was started and death was reversed. While part of the team applied external heart massage to supply circulation, Dr. Wigle set about to insert another electrode through a vein in his arm in order to restart the pacemaker that was keeping him alive.

Suddenly fibrillation set in. All activity promptly stopped while a defibrillator was put into position and two powerful electric shocks were sent through the convulsing heart. The heart began beating again at about twenty beats a minute but this was enough to give Dr. Wigle time to slip in the second wire and restore a normal beat.

Three weeks later, Mr. Outhouse was returned to surgery. This time the aortic valve was replaced and a permanent pacemaker installed. His eventual recovery was complete and he soon returned to his job as a TV repairman.

Most people think of heart attack as occurring in later life, most often to men past fifty. But heart trouble can threaten the life of children as well.

Four days before Christmas eight-year-old Nancy Hernandez along with a group of her schoolmates was admiring the beautiful Christmas tree and the lights at New York's Rockefeller Center. But suddenly the lights went out for Nancy: She became dizzy, her eyes rolled back in her head, and she fell unconscious to the ground. The attack was unprecedented. The little girl had not been ill although she had once fainted at home. In critical condition, Nancy was rushed by ambulance to St. Clare's hospital where three hours later her heart stopped beating. A team of doctors and nurses worked feverishly to bring her back. Nancy revived but in the next thirty hours she had *twenty* more heart arrests.

Top pediatricians took care of Nancy. When it was decided that she would need surgery she was moved to St. Vincent's Hospital and Medical Center. Here, a complete cardiac workup showed that she was the victim of a rare cardiac condition—a condition that is almost always fatal. For Nancy had a large hole between the small chambers of the heart as well as a heart blockage.

On February 15 a team of cardiac surgeons operated. For four hours the physicians worked, painstakingly repairing the large hole. A temporary pacemaker was implanted and kept connected for ten days after the operation. There were no precedents. In the past children suffering from this condition had died. But Nancy's heart didn't know that. Day by day it improved. As the weeks wore on and Nancy's health stabilized there was no doubt that she had made medical history.

Nancy was discharged from the hospital on March 4. When she told the doctors she wanted to be a ballerina, her physicians agreed that there was nothing to stop her, medically speaking. Nancy could live a normal life—play games, ride a bicycle, go swimming. For Nancy had a strong heartbeat which could take her through a long life.

Doctors are constantly innovating, improving, and adding to the weapons with which they fight death. In desperate cases, desperate measures are often undertaken.

When sixteen-year-old Bobby Munz was brought into New York's Mount Sinai Hospital on a hot August day recently, he was dying. A vicious virus infection, which had not responded to a wide battery of drugs, had blotted up most of the oxygen in his blood. Though a trachectomy was immediately performed to force oxygen into his lungs, Bobby continued to gasp for every breath, and turned blue. Bobby was resuscitated, but he needed further help. Dr. Julius H. Jacobson, director of the hospital's $800,000 hyperbatic oxygenation unit—a huge compression chamber, one of only three in the United States—was called into consultation.

Dr. Jacobson lost little time. He ordered that Bobby be placed immediately in the machine, though it had never been used in a case of this type.

"We have nothing to lose," he told his staff as Bobby was wheeled into the compression chamber. Atmospheric pressure was gradually increased to the equivalent of 35 feet below sea level. The aim was to force oxygen into the lungs and the bloodstream.

It was a long chance. What Dr. Jacobson was playing for, he explained, was time. If he could keep Bobby alive until the virus pneumonia, which was killing him, disappeared of its own account—as it usually does within a few days—they might be able to save him.

It worked. Bobby came out of the pressure chamber with more oxygen in his lungs and bloodstream and with enough strength to withstand the next few days. Once he was free of the virus, he was safe. From then on it was a question of re-building the six-foot-one-and-a-half-inch emaciated frame to the 170 pounds he normally carries.

Bobby came out of the hyperbatic unit not only with a chance to live, but with a brand-new plan of life. After seeing what medicine can do, Bobby decided he will be a doctor— a wish that his parents, Mr. and Mrs. Michael Munz of Long Beach, Long Island, hope to see come true.

6.
THE SCANDAL OF OUR EMERGENCY ROOMS

The thousands of men, women, and children seriously injured in life-threatening accidents can expect little help from the emergency medical systems that now exist throughout most of the United States. This is another reason why it is imperative for everyone to know how to administer modern resuscitative techniques.

Most of us blandly expect that when disaster strikes a doctor will treat us, an ambulance will arrive as soon as we call for one, and that we will receive expert care in a hospital. But the actual fact is that in many communities these essentials are not available when they are urgently needed.

In a few cities there are hospitals that practice resuscitative techniques routinely. With a trained and alerted staff and adequate equipment, they fight death—and often come out the victor. Firemen and policemen, as well as laymen who have had training in resuscitation, also play a valiant role in holding death at bay.

But in the large majority of our hospitals, the emergency room—long recognized as the weakest and most neglected department—has "only modest first-aid equipment" and is ill staffed to handle anything more than "minor conditions," in the opinion of the National Academy of Science. The American Heart Association estimates that fewer than half of our hospitals have staffs trained and equipped to give resuscitation. And it is to the emergency room that the maimed and the broken, the bruised and the battered victims of disaster are brought.

Yet in most emergency rooms even the severest cases are handled by interns who receive little instruction in emergency care as medical students. Surveys have revealed that hospitals are recurringly guilty of a variety of serious errors in treating patients, ranging from failure to promptly establish respiratory flow, to inappropriately administering narcotics and improperly evaluating a patient's condition!

In a Denver emergency room a check of the work of interns revealed that they gave inappropriate treatment in more than one out of five cases. And in only 5 percent of the cases did they establish the presence or absence of drug sensitivity before prescribing medication, despite the fact that drugs such as penicillin can be almost instantly fatal to patients allergic to them.

But untrained as they are, they are still superior *to the 78 percent of hospitals in this country that have no interns* and where for the most part nurses staff the emergency rooms. A number of studies have found that nurses "woefully lacking" in emergency training are often in complete charge, especially at night and on weekends, when at least half of all emergency cases arise and when staff doctors are likely to be absent. Courts are full of cases in which nurses have failed to recognize heart attacks and diabetic crises, have given incorrect medication that proved fatal, have left severely bleeding patients unattended and have administered injections so ineptly that the recipients were crippled for life.

Compounding the problems is a mushrooming demand for emergency-room care. Some forty million people will be flocking to the nation's hospitals this year in one form of "emergency" or another—almost three times as many as a decade ago. Many of the patients constituting this overtaxing burden come to the emergency room because they are unable to reach a doctor when they are in need of his services.

The inability to get a doctor even in the direst emergency

was underscored by two recent deaths that took place in Eliza-
beth, New Jersey. Both were attributed to heart attacks.

Police reported that Mrs. Leocadia Jaworski, a forty-three-
year-old housewife, died after they called ten doctors trying to
find one to treat her. James A. Reed, fifty-one, died an hour and
a half after police had begun the fruitless search for a doctor.

In a statewide survey conducted by the Michigan Blue
Cross in which researchers analyzed 3,650 case records of
patients who visited emergency rooms at twenty-two Michigan
hospitals during one week, it was found that 46 percent of the
patients came to the emergency room after unsuccessfully trying
to contact a doctor and 23 percent went straight to the hospital
because they did not think their doctor would be available. Almost one-third of the visits were made on Saturday or Sunday,
and 40 percent occurred on weekdays between 4 P.M. and 8 A.M.
when doctors are most difficult to reach. Unfortunately, it is
also the time when most emergencies arise.

In most cities the emergency rooms that provide basic
sources of care are crowded, uncomfortable, lacking in concern
for human dignity, and—to make it worse—no longer free. Yet
that is the best medical care available to millions of Americans.

The Blue Cross survey reveals that emergency rooms will
continue to become more and more crowded due to the natural
increase in the number of emergencies as a result of population
growth and shifts. Many families who move from city to city do
not have a family doctor. It is further estimated that in the near
future visits to emergency rooms across the country will reach
fifty million—more than double the number for 1960. By that
time officials believe emergency room visits may outnumber
regular hospital admissions.

The hectic arrival of patients with everything from a
bloodied nose to a massive heart attack would strain the facilities
of a well-run department. In most emergency rooms, understaffed and ill-equipped, the results are often tragic as patients in
desperate need of assistance are overlooked or kept waiting.

For example, in a crowded emergency room in a Chicago

hospital, a fifty-four-year-old man, his legs swollen, his skin gray and clammy, sat gasping for breath as he waited his turn. The young intern who was trying singlehandedly to take care of the constant surge of incoming patients was busy suturing a wound in an inner office.

Feeling nauseated, the man managed to stagger outside for some air. When he returned, the emergency room was more crowded than before. He found a seat and slumped into it, too weary to sit up. A few minutes later he appeared to go into a faint. No one paid any attention.

When the doctor finally made an appearance in the waiting room—he was trying to estimate how many serious cases awaited him—a woman sitting next to the man who "fainted," called him over.

"I think there is something wrong with this man," she told the doctor. There was, indeed. He was dead!

In Boston a seven-year-old who had fallen from the roof of a garage and been impaled on a picket fence which pierced his kidney lay on his mother's lap crying softly while he waited in hope of seeing a doctor. Before the boy's turn came he suffered a severe hemorrhage and died.

And in Cleveland a mother finding her fourteen-year-old son groggy and sick thought he was suffering from a virus. But when he became disoriented a suspicion that he might have taken an overdose of drugs caused her to bundle him into her car and drive to the nearest emergency room in hope of getting help. But the nurse in charge, harried and harassed, assured the mother there was nothing wrong with the boy. Without even taking his pulse or inquiring into his habits, she dismissed him. She suggested to the mother that if he wasn't any better the next day she bring her son to the afternoon clinic. But when the boy returned home he fell into a stuporous sleep from which he never woke.

Nor is the presence of a fully licensed physician certain comfort to an emergency patient. Many hospitals arbitrarily rotate their staff physicians to duty in the emergency department, regardless of their specialities. This can be dangerous to the patient, explains Dr. James Spencer, the Chicago surgeon who has campaigned nationally for improved emergency care. The victim of an automobile accident who has suffered multiple injuries, for example, needs the experience of someone other than an eye specialist involuntarily assigned to emergency duty. He might ignore important symptoms that would spell danger to a surgeon, easily missing a ruptured liver or prescribing the wrong care for a compound fracture.

A college football player with a broken leg was rushed to the emergency room at a Charleston, Illinois, hospital. The doctor in charge knew little about orthopedics. He applied a cast so tightly that it disrupted the boy's circulation to the extent that he eventually had to undergo amputation.

Sixteen-year-old Charles Ball, Jr., was one of four accident victims who were brought into the emergency room of a Memphis, Tennessee, hospital on a chilly October evening. The car in which Charles had been riding with his mother and two friends was struck broadside at an intersection, hurling him against an armrest. But because Charles had no visible injuries he was left without care while the nurses and intern worked on his bleeding companions.

Ignored and in shock Charles lay on a stretcher. When the pain became too much to bear he tried to get help. But when he tried to groggily get to his feet a uniform watchman shoved him down and admonished him not to be a nuisance. Groaning, Charles doubled his knees to his chest. A passing intern stopped long enough to scrawl on a record: "Very unruly—appears intoxicated." The fact was that Charles had never had a drink in his life. An excellent student, he and his mother were returning from a church benefit when the accident occurred.

Charles tried again to get up but was quickly wrestled down by nurses and ambulance attendants who flipped him onto his stomach. A guard sat across his feet; another planted his knees in the small of the boy's back.

From where she lay in a curtained cubicle nearby, Charles's

injured mother could hear him scream, "Please don't! Stop! You're killing me!"

Furious at the commotion, the intern ordered that the boy be lashed to his stretcher and transferred to a municipal hospital that "handles drunks."

In the ambulance when Charles's knees folded up again, the watchman yanked his legs straight. In that moment vast quantities of blood in the body of Charles Ball, Jr., poured into his abdominal cavity. In the crash his liver had been severely lacerated. His writhing movements were desperate attempts to lessen the excruciating pain. As the ambulance, siren shrieking, careened away, Charles Ball, who was being forcibly held down, died.

An expert medical witness later testified that a "very short examination," even simple blood-pressure checks, would have promptly revealed Charles's internal crisis. Instead, the neglect and rough handling prompted by an inexperienced young doctor's offhand "diagnosis" destroyed whatever clotting had taken place, intensified the hidden bleeding—and lost a life that quite possibly could have been saved.

Ignorance is often accompanied by poor equipment and unsanitary conditions. In a survey of New York hospitals it was discovered that many of the large municipal institutions, that serve thousands of patients, lacked life-saving resuscitators respirators, defibrillators, electrocardiograph machines or suitable drugs in their emergency rooms. Doctors staffing the emergency quarters admitted they often lost patients because they lacked the proper equipment to treat them. Other hospitals in the group were filthy and were termed "fire traps" when the investigators found them minus sprinkler systems and with their fire hoses not connected to any water source.

Testifying before a State Investigating Commission in March, 1968, doctors told of conditions in hospitals that were reminiscent of the dark ages. Dr. Samuel H. Rubin, Chief of Medicine at Metropolitan Hospital and professor of medicine at New York Medical College, testified that many patients who are critically ill are doomed to die because there were not enough X-ray machines to make diagnoses. "We're missing cancers and we're missing ulcers because patients have to wait two to three months before an X ray is taken," stated Dr. Rubin. The one-thousand-bed municipal hospital, he said, had only four X-ray machines, one of which was usually broken—equipment that might suffice for a two-hundred-bed hospital.

Many of the patients, after being rebuffed time and again in the emergency room, don't bother to come back to the hospital, the doctor said. "They live with their own pain and enter the hospital months later with extensive metastasis [malignancy]. They die soon afterwards."

Dr. Edward D. Coates, assistant director of the New York office of the State Health Department, testifying before the commission, told of two patients dying at Coney Island Medical Hospital while awaiting treatment in the emergency room.

"One of the patients, a heart attack victim, needed extremely prompt attention," said Dr. Coates. "But he had to wait three hours. He was dead by the time help was available."

Miss Lucille Frank, supervisor of the emergency room and Intensive Care Unit at Coney Island Hospital until she quit in November, 1967, bemoaned the intolerable conditions that existed. There was scarcity of such vital equipment as stretchers, respirators, suction machines, examining tables, and fresh linens. Miss Frank told of a patient suffering from heat prostration brought into the sweltering emergency room. "I took the fan off the wall and set it up in front of him with a bag of ice cubes," she said. It was the best she could do under the circumstances.

Nor are the municipal hospitals the only guilty ones. A surprise visit by an investigating committee to a four-hundred-bed voluntary hospital in Manhattan—maintained by voluntary contributions from the public—disclosed that the emergency room had no life-saving equipment. A spokesman for the hospital later insisted that the necessary equipment was elsewhere in the building. Two young interns interviewed by a newspaper reporter admitted that patients often died because it took too long to get the equipment to the emergency quarters.

New York is not unique in this respect. In a statewide survey of Colorado hospitals, whose results, the AMA says, "could easily be transferred to any region in the country," investigators found that nearly one out of three emergency rooms lacked necessary medications, artificial breathing apparatus, cardiac equipment, and suction machines. And the procedures for handling antiseptics, used in treating a high percentage of emergency patients, were found to be "unscientific, illogical, and improperly organized" in the majority of hospitals.

The inadequate care facilities and insufficiently trained personnel take their toll. A heart attack patient rushed to the emergency room of a community hospital in California recently began receiving immediate emergency treatment. Scarcely ten minutes later, a far more serious heart case was wheeled in. Because the emergency room had only enough equipment to handle one patient, hospital attendants were forced to transfer their efforts to the new arrival.

After an hour's work, the emergency room personnel were able to send the second patient to intensive care, and return to the first arrival. But the hour's lapse had changed the favorable situation. The first patient had lost ground during the long wait. He died in the emergency room.

In a Chicago hospital the door to the emergency room is locked at night—the very time when emergencies are most apt to occur. The ambulance attendants have to ring a doorbell and wait for the night supervisor to come along and open the door. In inclement weather, or when the patient is critically ill, the wait can prove fatal.

In another Chicago hospital the entrance to the emergency room is via a tedious labyrinth. After arriving at the hospital the patient is taken to a basement in one elevator, transported down a corridor to another elevator, then taken up to the third floor where the emergency room is located.

Often the hospital administrator refuses to admit the patient. During a busy late afternoon on a Friday in February, 1968, Philip Johnston was rushing his wife, who was in advanced labor, to Columbus Hospital on Chicago's Near North Side. But before they could reach the hospital, Mrs. Johnston gave birth to their fourth child on the front seat of their car.

Frantic, Johnston hailed a patrolman. Sirens howling and lights flashing, the policeman's squad car led the couple and their newborn daughter to the nearest hospital, the ninety-six-bed Clark Street unit of the Sheridan General Hospital. There, the policeman rushed into the hospital and blurted out the problem. Without even glancing at the mother and child in the Johnston car, a staff physician turned them away and sent them to Edgewater Hospital, a larger facility about a mile and a half away. When the Johnstons finally arrived at Edgewater, the infant was not breathing. Although mouth-to-mouth resuscitation revived her, the baby girl died twenty-one hours later.

The callousness of the doctor who refused admission to the woman and infant, and the resulting death of the child, aroused public ire when the story broke in the newspapers. Mayor Richard J. Daley ordered an immediate investigation. A series of public hearings were held and testimony taken from all the principals—all except the physician involved. He disappeared when it became known that, though he had represented himself as a graduate of the Medical School of the National University of Mexico in Mexico City, he was not licensed in Illinois and had not been certified by the Educational Council for Foreign Medical Graduates. He failed on four successive occasions to qualify in the examinations for foreign medical graduates. This seemed to underscore the existing situation in emergency rooms.

After the investigation, the city of Chicago ordered the badly understaffed and poorly run Sheridan General Hospital to shut down and issued orders that all patients be transferred to other institutions.

In many cities patients in critical conditions are often moved from a private hospital to a large public institution because the first hospital decides that the patient will be unable to pay his bill or that it will be paid—only after long delays—by the welfare department. Many of the transfers are carried out under unsafe conditions, says Dr. Donald Kozoll, Director of Admissions at Chicago's Cook County Hospital. He told of a middle-aged woman in coma, a man in the throes of a heart attack, a young man with a collapsed lung, and a fourteen-year-old boy whose broken ankle had been put in a cast without being set—all were trundled across the city unattended by medical personnel.

The dire results that often ensue when inexperienced, indifferent doctors take it upon themselves to transfer critically ill patients, were revealed by Dr. Robert J. Freeark, Chief of Surgury at Cook County. He cited the case of a man who crashed into a light pole and was taken by a fire department ambulance to the 150-bed Belmont Community Hospital. A house physician there stitched up several facial lacerations, decided that the man had a fractured thigh and a probable fractured jaw, but took no X rays. He then transferred the patient to Cook County Trauma Center.

He was admitted to Cook County Hospital more than two hours after the accident in a state of deep shock, says Dr. Freeark. An abdominal puncture revealed that the patient's peritoneal cavity was filled with blood from a severely ruptured liver. He died on the operating table.

In a letter to a Chicago newspaper, Dr. Freeark blamed the patient's death on the lack of a citywide plan for the care of the acutely injured. A Chicago newspaper columnist summed up the situation succinctly: "Now that the doctors seem to be solving the problem of transplant rejection, they had better get to work on the patient rejection problem."

The inescapable conclusion of the foregoing events and related statistics is that widespread apathy among both laymen and professionals has left emergency care a century behind the times.

7.
LIVES IMPERILED BY AMBULANCE SERVICES

All too often a ride in an ambulance is anything but life-saving. Inadequate as our emergency rooms are, nationwide surveys demonstrate that the ambulance service available in most cities and suburban areas is even more perilous. Ambulances exist in our country in the frightening ratio of one per five thousand persons. The surveys show the wait for an ambulance is often one and sometimes as many as five hours. *And 72 percent of the calls for ambulances are never answered.*

In many communities a dilapidated station wagon is used as an ambulance without being equipped with as much as a Band-Aid. And there are many towns and suburban areas that have no ambulance service whatsoever.

In 1969, according to the National Safety Council, there were approximately eleven million disabling accidents in the United States. A great many of the victims traveled to the hospital by ambulance—an experience that was almost as bad as the accident.

It was raining—one of the hard rains that often breaks the Florida mid-day heat—when Ed Bagely came out of the building where his office was located. A robust young man, Ed walked briskly towards a restaurant on the next block. He had almost reached his destination when he was struck by a truck that suddenly backed out of an alley.

The policeman on the beat knew Ed, as did several of the men who came running out of nearby offices. Ed was conscious but his breathing had a harsh rasp and his face had the gray, clammy look that indicated he was in shock. He needed medical care quickly.

The policeman covered Ed with his own raincoat and rushed to a phone to call an ambulance. While Ed Bagely, who was bleeding internally, went into deeper shock, the policeman made more than a dozen calls before he finally located an ambulance.

The contraption that finally arrived at the scene of the accident was a converted station wagon with a wheeled cot. The only attendant was the driver. There was no emergency medical equipment, nor anyone to administer any kind of first aid.

Sirens wailing and lights flashing, the ambulance sped to the hospital while Ed slowly bled to death. The emergency physician pronounced him dead on arrival.

The doctor who saw Ed looked angry and frustrated. "There's nothing we can do now," he said. "But if there had been competent emergency treatment in the ambulance he would have reached us alive and we could have saved him."

Tragically, this is not an isolated case. Similar incidents occur every day throughout the nation. According to Dr. Charles C. Edwards, Director of the American Medical Association's Division of Socio-Economic Activities: "A soldier wounded in the jungle of Vietnam often gets quicker and more comprehensive emergency care than an accident victim on the highway." Due primarily to the speed with which casualties are given medical attention on the battlefield, the mortality rate of the wounded who die after entering medical channels is less than 1 percent. (This compares with 2.2 percent in the Korean War, 4.5 percent in World War II, and 8.5 percent in World War 1.)

Many of the 60,485 persons not killed outright who died during the year 1969 as a result of vehicular accidents never reached hospitals. Often they died at the scene of the accident because ambulances took too long in arriving and didn't give the injured the care they needed either there or during transport to the hospital.

Dr. Richard Manegold, emergency expert of the American Medical Association, recently pointed out that 70 percent of the deaths occurred in rural areas. He said: "In general, the accidents producing these deaths were not as severe as those in urban areas. It is the time element in getting help to them that accounts for the morbid statistics."

The chief and often the only qualification for many ambulance attendants is that they have a driver's license. "Yet they must frequently make vital decisions," says Dr. Manegold. "Should a patient with a broken back be moved? Is mouth-to-mouth respiration needed? Is the patient in shock? Can bleeding be controlled? Unless ambulance drivers understand such things, a life that might be saved is lost."

"In most regions, attendants on the ambulance that answers your emergency call are likely to be as untrained as they are ill equipped," says Francis Keppel, former Assistant Secretary of the Department of Health, Education and Welfare. He has charged that "for the most part" ambulance attendants "don't know a tourniquet from a squash racket, much less how to move a person with an injured back or how to treat for shock." Surveys have found that in some states—North Dakota and Missouri, for example—as few as one-fourth of the ambulance attendants are trained in first aid. In Chicago, the only "equipment" some private ambulances carry for handling psychotic patients is a blackjack.

One emergency case out of every three, according to one national survey, is in some way mishandled, and in some states public health officials suspect that, in the category of rural auto accidents alone, "at least one-half of the deaths need not occur."

"Thousands die every year because of deficiencies in our emergency medical service. Thousands of others are condemned to wheel chairs or crutches for life," says Dr. Robert H. Kennedy, a New York surgeon recognized as the nation's foremost authority on emergency care. "The figures would be even higher if emergencies arising from sudden illness are included."

In a large southern city a teen-age girl, pinned in a car after a major but nonfatal accident, was extracted by the police and ambulance personnel on the scene. The two ambulance attendants applied splints to the girl's shattered leg and loaded her into their $15,000 ambulance.

Unfortunately, neither of the attendants was trained sufficiently to realize that the splints they applied caused the bone slivers in the girl's leg to sever tendons and nerves necessary for locomotion. The girl will walk again, but she will always have a noticeable limp—a limp she could have been spared if proper emergency measures had been taken.

The estimated forty thousand ambulances in this country are operated by a bewildering and uncoordinated welter of agencies, including mortuaries, hospitals, fire and police departments, private firms, and volunteer rescue squads. Undertakers operate more of the nation's ambulances (over 50 percent) than any other group. This is particularly true in rural America and small towns, a tradition that began in the days when the undertaker was the only person in town with a suitable vehicle.

According to Dr. Kennedy, who has conducted an intensive investigation for the American College of Surgeons, undertakers provide some of the worst service. The attendants of these vehicles more often resemble ghouls than rescuers. Considering that funerals are far more lucrative than transporting a live patient in urgent need of medical care, there is an overwhelming temptation for operators of ambulance-hearses to concentrate on bodies instead of live victims. Police officials have told medical assemblies that they frequently see injured persons ignored at accident scenes while mortuary ambulance attendants scramble to pick up the dead.

In some cases, says Dr. Kennedy, state laws demanding that the injured be removed first "have been enforced at gunpoint." In one city, when three competing funeral-home ambulances arrived at an accident to find one person dead and two badly injured, police had to break up a fist fight among the ambulance operators over who would take the dead man.

Dr. Manegold points out that live passengers present to mortuary personnel a terrible conflict of interest: "Should we give the victim artificial respiration and take him to the hospital, or let him die en route and take him to the funeral home?"

Other ambulance personnel undoubtedly are harassed by the same question. For instance in Chicago, attendants for private firms reportedly can collect $50 "tips" from funeral homes for the bodies of patients who die in ambulances.

"Picture yourself," says a newsman who exposed this situation, "being rushed to the hospital, and the 'concerned' ambulance driver hoping you won't make it."

Dr. Charles Voorhis, of Kent, Ohio, writing in the *AMA Journal,* tells of seeing "unconscious patients brought into the emergency room face down on the ambulance stretcher" or "suffocating under blankets." Often, he says, a patient arrives with the oxygen mask over his face filled with "blood and vomitus," effectively preventing him from getting air.

Such abuses have arisen in an almost universal climate of official apathy toward ambulance practices declares Dr. Kennedy. Paradoxically, beauticians, barbers, and a host of other nonmedical personnel must be licensed and regulated in most states. Nonetheless, according to the Ambulance Association of America, only sixteen states have standards for equipment or attendant-training in the private ambulance industry, which daily is confronted with life-or-death situations.

Colorado investigators disclosed in 1967 that 80 percent of the state's ambulance operators give no evidence of using disinfectants to clean equipment, even after transporting infectious patients.

In North Carolina half the services checked in 1965 did not even use soap and water and some did not bother to change stretcher linens. More than half of the ambulances in the state lacked such essential items as splints, bandages, oxygen tanks, portable resuscitators. And only a minority of ambulances had flares, two-way radios, and fire extinguishers. Fully 29 percent of ambulance operators in the state had no first-aid training. And even where personnel did have some training, they could not always administer to the patient on the way to the hospital, for 26 percent of all ambulance units sent only a driver on a call.

But even in cities where most of the ambulances are modern and well equipped and the personnel is trained in life-saving, there is no guarantee that you'll get the care you need when you need it. In Brooklyn, New York, a pedestrian was hit by a car at an intersection. The police arrived quickly and put in repeated calls for an ambulance. But Kings County Hospital—a mere eight blocks and five minutes away. from the scene—had more calls than it could handle and was unable to respond for more than an hour.

In busy Manhattan an average of one thousand calls a day pour in for police-dispatched ambulances, with peak loads so far beyond capacity, according to one investigation, that even fire victims sometimes wait thirty minutes for help, often with fatal results.

In Nevada, where equipment is sparsely distributed and only a minority of ambulance services are ready to roll twenty-four hours a day, more than one-third require an average of longer than an hour to bring a patient to a hospital.

In Phoenix, Arizona, an ambulance service confronted with an out-of-town emergency call took two hours to reach a middle-aged farm worker who lived only twenty miles out of the city. He was suffering mysterious stomach pains when the call for the ambulance was put in. When it arrived, he was dead.

Yet, paradoxically, once the ambulances have a patient in tow, there is a reckless addiction to speed. In a rural community in North Dakota, a woman who became seriously ill after giving birth was dispatched by ambulance to a hospital in Bismarck, ninety miles away. Her husband went along. Speeding over the crest of a hill, the ambulance crashed into a farm truck. Both wife and husband were killed, as was the ambulance driver.

In Kansas City, Missouri, an ambulance carrying a young woman badly hurt in an auto accident rocketed through the downtown section and collided with a passenger car. The accident sent four more victims to the hospital, including the ambulance driver.

Ironically, studies have proven that undue speed is rarely necessary in ambulance runs. In an analysis of 2,500 emergency trips in Flint, Michigan, Drs. George J. Curry and Sydney N. Lyttle reported that speed—defined as going sixty rather than thirty miles an hour—would not have benefited a single patient. In fact, in nine of the accident cases, the doctors reported "a wild, weaving, siren-screeching ride to the hospital probably was responsible for death or permanent invalidism. These included seven cases of multiple rib fractures and two fracture dislocations of the cervical spine.

When Medicare became effective in July, 1966, some observers hoped that abuses in emergency medical care would be alleviated. To qualify for Medicare payments, ambulances were to maintain twenty-four-hour service, carry oxygen, as well as unspecified "first aid supplies," and at least one attendant with the equivalent of advanced Red Cross first-aid instruction. Emergency rooms were to assure "prompt" diagnosis and treatment, see that "adequate" medical and nursing personnel were on duty or on call at all times, arrange for all patients to see a doctor, and keep appropriate medical records.

Some ambulance companies, however, went out of business rather than conform—as others did during 1968 because of new federal wage regulations. Others simply refused to handle Medicare patients. A great many joined hospitals in strong protests over the cost of improving their operations.

As a result, says Dr. James Spencer, the Chicago surgeon, government enforcement of the regulations has been "lenient," and the Medicare Act, despite its potential "has not to date had any appreciable effect" on emergency service. In addition, many experts are convinced the law's provisions are so vague and minimal that even if adhered to they do not fill the gaping void in emergency care.

Ambulance personnel should "undergo extensive instruction," says Dr. Sam F. Seeley, emergency care expert for the National Research Council. "They treat seriously injured accident victims under emergency conditions and they should be given particularly rigorous training."

Dr. J. D. Farrington, chairman of the subcommittee on transportation of American College of Surgeons' Committee on Trauma, believes that instruction in basic anatomy and physiology should be mandatory for all ambulance personnel. Emergency care should include giving fluids to shock patients, for example, and performing external cardiac compression. "An ambulance attendant should know enough medicine to meaningfully treat the entire patient in the emergency, not just one or two elements of his problem. And he should be impressed with the fact that his work is critical."

There is no mystery about running a decent ambulance service; the same basic ingredients are required in both urban and rural areas. The various authorities—the American College of Surgeons, the U.S. Public Health Service, the National Safety Council—agree that the necessary elements are: (1) an adequate number of vehicles properly maintained and safely driven; (2) speedy communications, with a central location to receive all ambulance calls and two-way radio contact with each ambulance; (3) an ample supply of first-aid equipment on each vehicle; (4) well-trained personnel.

All that remains is to put such a service into action.

Dr. Peter Safar, of Pittsburgh's University-Presbyterian Hospital, who is internationally known as an expert in emergency care, has urged a sweeping revision of our present-day emergency system. Pointing out that the number of possible deaths reversible by modern respiration and cardiac resuscitation exceeds that of many infectious diseases, Dr. Safar makes it clear that we will be able to effectively turn back death only if we have an *improved community-wide emergency care organization that is far more resuscitation-oriented than at present.*

Dr. Safar cites the three aspects of emergency care essential to good results:

The thorough knowledge of modern resuscitative techniques by the public at large. This means men, women, and teen-agers will have training in the art of resuscitation; that the techniques will have been implanted in grade schools and continued through high school; that special classes will be available for men and women who wish to learn how to perform the modern techniques that can play a vital role in reversing death.

Reorganization of our ambulance service. This includes the establishment of minimal standards for personal training of ambulance personnel, adequate equipment available on each ambulance, and a central ambulance dispatching system that will make an ambulance available in the shortest possible time after death strikes.

Upgrading of hospital emergency room care. This calls for coverage around the clock by physicians experienced in the art of resuscitation. Acute life-threatening conditions in emergency room admissions include airway obstruction, pulselessness, unconsciousness, respiratory distress, massive hemorrhage, head injury, and crushing injury of the chest. Mortality from these injuries could be greatly reduced if modern resuscitative techniques were immediately and skillfully applied.

Specialists who have made a study of unexpected death in this country feel that a dramatic educational drive aimed at both the medical profession and the public is needed if we are to awaken people to the life-saving possibilities of the new resuscitation techniques.

That public interest and community participation can completely change the status of emergency care, upgrading it to the point where loss of life is drastically cut, has been proven by the few towns and cities where citizens have taken an active interest in reorganizing their emergency care systems.

Typical of what citizens can do is the case of Summit, New Jersey, where a volunteer first-aid squad of businessmen and housewives run an ambulance service. All participants take special training in emergency procedures, and like volunteer groups in other small towns are highly motivated.

In its first three months of operation the Summit group successfully handled more than one hundred cases. Since then its skill has continued to save lives. One such case involved a critically ill librarian who was hospitalized in Summit with bronchial pneumonia. He had previously undergone open-heart surgery at a hospital in Washington, D.C., and the Summit doctors believed that he should be treated there. The volunteers quickly rigged up a special oxygen system and arranged a state-by-state escort for their ambulance. In just four hours, they safely delivered the patient free of charge.

"He was very fortunate," an observer noted later, "to get sick in Summit."

The American College of Surgeons rates the volunteer service of Greenport in upstate New York as one of the best in the country. Greenport is one of ten towns in Columbia County that supports voluntary ambulance services. Each town has its own ambulances, purchased with funds raised by dances, raffles, parties, and door-to-door soliciting. Trained to meet any emergency, the rescue squads of the county, which number two hundred volunteers, often pool their resources when a large disaster erupts in any part of the county.

On the evening of September 10, 1963, Memorial Hospital in Greenport was notified that two people had been hurt in a train accident. An ambulance left immediately. But on arrival at the scene the ambulance attendants saw that a train had collided with a switch engine, and many more were injured. A great many ambulances would be needed. Within minutes the alarm had gone out to the county and ambulances began streaming to Greenport from every township—each manned by trained volunteers. The Mutual Aid Plan developed by the volunteers was working perfectly. Within an hour twenty-four injured passengers had been rushed to Memorial Hospital and were receiving treatment.

Three members of one family owe their lives to the immediate help offered by the Greenport rescue squad. One night a telephone operator at Memorial Hospital in Greenport heard a voice say, "Get an ambulance out to the Brown residence . . . hurry . . . coal gas . . . help please . . . hurry or you'll be too late."

The voice became faint and trailed off as the man at the other end collapsed. The call was made by twenty-three-year-old Gordon Evans. He was trying to force out further information when his strength gave out.

But even while Evans was on the wire another telephone operator had started rounding up members of the Greenport rescue squad. Fortunately for Evans, John Zlomeck, Clinton Stickles, and Andrea Hart, Jr., had just brought in a highway accident case. They returned to their ambulance, equipped with the very latest medical paraphernalia, and were off. Meanwhile, the operator alerted the town's second ambulance crew of the emergency, for no one knew how many people were involved.

The crew of the first ambulance found the house locked, but through a window the men could see young Evans, unconscious on the floor, the telephone still in his hand. They smashed a door, rushed in and carried Evans out into the fresh air. Two of the men started immediate resuscitation. They had no way of knowing whether anyone else was trapped in the gas-filled home, but their training demanded that they make a thorough search.

In the bedroom Zlomeck found the body of Mrs. Eleanor Evans, forty-nine-year-old mother of Gordon Evans, and in the kitchen they found his grandmother, seventy-six-year-old Nellie Brown. Quickly both women were carried out. The second ambulance had arrived by this time, thus permitting six trained rescue workers to apply resuscitation to the unconscious victims.

"It didn't look at all good," Stickles recalled. "We had four small tanks and one large tank of oxygen which we forced into their lungs. We used every resuscitation trick we knew. But it was forty-five minutes before any of them responded."

Only when voluntary breathing was established were the victims placed in ambulances. With resuscitation continuing, they were raced to the hospital. All three made a complete recovery thanks to the immediate assistance they received. Doctors who cared for the victims were frank in saying that another five minutes would have been fatal.

All the ambulance volunteers of Columbia County are trained by the American Red Cross. They give thousands of hours each year to provide prompt emergency care for the county's population of forty thousand people, as well as the thousands of motorists on the highways that crisscross the county. It is difficult to estimate just how many calls are answered by the combined crews but in the year 1967 the ambulance teams of Greenport answered 1,514 calls.

The ambulance volunteers receive periodic retraining by the Red Cross in order that they employ at all times the latest resuscitative techniques. So that they are ready for anything, the volunteers, with four doctors supervising, stage mock disasters. Each squad is assigned a group of patients to care for and transport. They must be able to splint, bandage, give oxygen, stop bleeding, do closed-heart massage, and give mouth-to-mouth resuscitation. The doctors check the patients and point out mistakes that are made. For the most part, however, the physicians are high in their praise, for the ambulance drivers are dedicated men, and are very careful of how they treat patients.

The death of a stranger triggered the formation of a new mobile emergency service in Southern California that is helping others to survive. The man, a visitor in Rancho Santa Fe, was taking a walk when he was suddenly stricken by a heart attack.

Moaning, he fell to the ground. Two men heard him, and ran
to give assistance. One started artificial respiration while the
other raced to a telephone to notify the fire department. Both
a doctor and an ambulance were summoned.

Dr. Quentin L. Wood reached the patient in ten minutes. The
ambulance arrived fifteen minutes later. Thirty minutes after the
ambulance arrived, the man was admitted to Scripps Hospital in
San Diego, which has a Coronary Care Unit—a type of specialized hospital care that is drastically reducing the deaths of heart
patients across the country. But it was too late for the stranger.
He died twenty minutes after admission.

Dr. Wood was oppressed by the feeling that something was
terribly wrong. In one of the richest communities in California,
a man had died because the special kind of aid he needed was not
available to him in time to save his life. If the Coronary Care
Unit could have been moved to the patient, he could have been
saved. Dr. Wood decided "We are doing things backwards."
Treatment should be rushed to the patient, not the patient to
the treatment. Out of this profound thought has grown a service
that is unique in this country.

Dr. Wood conferred with prominent citizens of the community about his idea—an ambulance that would be in reality a
small hospital on wheels, one which could be rushed to any
victim who needed immediate help. There was an enthusiastic
response from the community.

Retired Fire Commissioner Leon Janinet, who had seen
many a man die because he did not receive proper help in time,
underwrote the cost of the vehicle. This meant no time would
be lost in taking up contributions and the project could go into
swift action.

The next big decision was to pick a vehicle that would
serve the desired purpose. It had to be sturdy enough to navigate
back roads, and it needed to be spacious. The committee—which
included Dr. Wood, Fire Chief James A. Fox of Rancho Sante
Fe, as well as Mr. Janinet—finally settled on a Chevrolet van,

equipped with large balloon tires on the rear wheels for easy riding.

The van was finished with a smooth interior of wood and metal that could easily be kept clean. Shallow cabinets were built to one side. All equipment was movable—for use outside the ambulance as well as inside. A comfortable cushioned seat near the head of the table that occupied the center of the ambulance enabled the doctor or an attendant to remain beside the patient when not working over him. Hooks at the side were strong enough to support two additional stretchers if required. An outside compartment over the rear wheels held an extra oxygen supply.

But it was the electronic equipment that was unique. For this ambulance was designed to give the kind of intensive care that is usually provided in hospital coronary care units. There was a monitor that would give the physician a minute-by-minute report of the heart's action, an electrocardiograph, a resuscitator to take over the task of breathing for the patient, and a defibrillator that could be used to shock the fibrillating heart back to normal rhythm. A coronary patient in desperate need of help would have this equipment brought to his side and he would receive intensive care on the spot.

There was also equipment for giving intravenous infusions, blood plasma, a suction machine, splints, bandages, suturing equipment, and a full compartment of necessary medications—all of them vitally important in treating emergency patients.

The town's residents paid for all the equipment. The ambulance would function as a small hospital able to provide treatment not only to heart patients but stroke victims, those suffering collapse of any kind, hemorrhaging, obstetrical emergencies, allergic reactions, and fractures. None of these could afford to wait for the ambulance to take a long trip to the hospital. Some of the patients—if they received proper treatment by ambulance personnel—might be able to return to their homes instead of a hospital.

Before the ambulance was put into operation all attendants received training courses under the direction of the Red Cross. A physician would always ride the ambulance when it answered a disaster call. The new vehicle has no sirens, no flashing lights, for the doctors felt that an accident victim, a heart attack patient, or an acutely ill person does not need a frenzied, clanging ride. What he must have is tranquility, reassurance, and care. A speaking tube, which is also the horn, acts as a warning to those on the road. Drivers of the vehicles are instructed to use a low but audible voice as they announce: "Please clear the road; this is an emergency vehicle."

The hospital on wheels went on duty August 27, 1967—exactly one year after the stranger died in Rancho Sante Fe because proper help did not reach him in time. It now is always on twenty-four-hour alert.

An ambulance similarly equipped and manned by two doctors is now being dispatched from St. Vincent's Hospital in New York City. The hospital ambulance, which covers the lower part of Manhattan, was made possible by an $88,000 grant from the New York Regional Program (a federal project that seeks to close the gap between new medical discoveries and their delivery to people whose lives depend on them).

In the first two months of operation the St. Vincent's heart squad saved more than 90 percent of the heart victims it treated on the spot.

"For the patient experiencing a first heart attack the first sixty minutes are critical," says Dr. William J. Grace, Chief of Medicine at St. Vincent's. "If we can get him by then, chances are we can save him."

Other cities such as Flint, Michigan, and Miami, Florida, have reasoned that emergency transportation is as vital a part of public service as fire and police protection and, therefore, have granted annual subsides to private ambulance firms, enabling them to upgrade employees and facilities. Still others, such as Louisville, Baltimore, and San Francisco, have made ambulance operation a responsibility of local fire, police, or health departments.

As for the emergency room difficulties, they lie, for the most part, in the lack of trained medical men to handle the large influx of patients. Physicians who practice regularly in hospital emergency rooms need special training to meet the many varied and often desperate situations that routinely present themselves, asserts Dr. Reinald Leidelmeyer, co-chairman of the Emergency Room department at Fairfax Hospital in Falls Church, Virginia. Because the doctor in the emergency room must "treat patients he has never seen before for any ailment or injury," his training must be in the emergency room just as surely as the surgeon's must be in the operating room.

Says Dr. Leidelmeyer: "He must know how to handle medical equipment—how to set up cardiac resuscitation apparatus and which button to push on the defibrillator. He's got to be able to perform a tracheotomy, to put in a chest drain, and to know what to do in cases of poisoning. He's got to have enough psychiatric experience to spot and deal with real psychotics. And he has to know how to manage alcoholics brought into the emergency room.

"No average doctor knows how to handle all these things. That is why specialized training is necessary for ER work and why such work must be, and I believe soon will be, recognized as a specialty. Because every doctor is called on to deal with an emergency at some time, interns should be routinely rotated through the emergency rooms."

A survey made recently by the Michigan Blue Cross Association revealed that some hospitals are experimenting quite successfully with the employment of a group of qualified physicians to staff the emergency room on a full-time basis.

Typical of how emergency care can be put on a sound basis is the situation in Alexandria, Virginia, a rambling bedroom city for Washington, D.C., with a population of 117,000, housing mostly government employees.

Six years ago the emergency room in Alexandria's only hospital was stuck away in the basement. Patients had to wait in a corridor and complained bitterly about long delays in obtaining treatment or of being brusquely dismissed if their illnesses or injuries didn't appear serious enough to merit treatment. The emergency staff consisted of nurses who generally urged patients to wait until their family physician could take care of the emergency.

Serving on a staff committee studying the problem, Dr. James D. Mills, Jr., a general practioner for seven years, suggested that the emergency service be viewed as a full-time "specialty" similar to other branches of medicine. To man the emergency service around the clock, Dr. Mills recruited three of his colleagues. Meanwhile, part of the ground floor was completely renovated to accommodate a four-room emergency department, as well as separate waiting room and staff offices. One room is reserved for cardiac cases, another for trauma, a third for gynecology and obstetrics, a fourth for illness and infections. Modern equipment is used for a multitude of common contingencies.

During unusually busy periods the doctors call on military physicians from nearby veterans hospitals to help out, and they consult appropriate specialists about complicated cases. The physicians, all of whom have ten-year contracts with the hospital, bill the patients directly and make as much—or more—than they did in private practice.

Another hospital which has "farmed out" professional services in its emergency rooms is the Miami Valley Hospital, in Dayton, Ohio. The emergency department, which handles about forty thousand patients a year, has three full-time and two part-time doctors who provide twenty-four-hour coverage on a fee-for-service basis. But these progressive areas are pitifully few.

Mayor John Lindsay of New York, recently addressing ten thousand volunteer workers, made the point that "people

power humanizes government." New legislation and new procedures that improve conditions in a community are often the
result of lay people making their needs known—and insisting
that constructive action be taken.

8.

NEW EMERGENCY SYSTEMS

The entire emergency situation has been characterized by doctors and government officials as itself being an emergency on a national scale. So poor is the function of our emergency departments—which today affect the lives of more citizens than any other medical facility—that it has aroused the concern and dismay of everyone from former President Lyndon Johnson to the leaders of such nationally known medical groups as the American Medical Association, the American Heart Association, and the U.S. Public Health Department.

To overcome the shocking conditions that typify this situation a number of plans have been put before the public. In a special message to Congress on March 4, 1968, former President Johnson proposed a $15.6 billion "Health in America" program outlining five major health goals: to curb infant mortality, provide more health personnel, combat soaring medical costs, *lower accident deaths*, and *seek volunteer efforts by doctors, hospitals, and others to provide better health for all Americans.*

The former President pointed out that over the last fifty years the accident category has risen from twenty-eighth on the list of causes of death to fourth.

A new pilot plan now being tested in three Philadelphia hospitals—Jefferson Medical College, Hahnemann Medical College, and Pennsylvania University—has tackled the emergency difficulties with such modern devices as computers, helicopters, and automatic alert systems. The plan is demonstrating that the dangerous time lag in bringing a patient together with life-saving equipment and doctors, which is maddening to medical men and sometimes fatal to their patients, can be solved.

With the aid of a Public Health Service grant and a computer, Dr. Joel Nobel, who heads a Research Center on Emergency Care—the only one in the country—working with systems engineer Richard M. Rauch mathematically simulated all the activities going on during a typical emergency. They even included the speed with which a nurse can push an emergency cart. They checked their computer findings by conducting drills and clocking every step.

The result was Dr. Nobel's Area-Wide Emergency Medical System—known as AEMS—which encompasses all available facilities of the community. Dr. Nobel points out that many of the techniques, systems, and skills required to save lives are already accessible. What is needed is to put them all together and make them work.

One of the major problems in emergency care is communications. The majority of cities do not have central communication centers to dispatch ambulances and other emergency equipment to the scene of the disaster or to allocate hospital beds in the area.

The AEMS system makes use of the Philadelphia Fire Department's computer for this purpose. Dr. Nobel points out that most large cities have traffic computers that could be utilized to direct emergency care.

The dispatching center takes into account such factors as emergency room loads, physical availability, bed space, special facilities such as burn units or coronary care units. The computer directs the appropriate emergency conveyance—ambulance, helicopter, or boat—to pick up the patient. It also selects the hospital best situated to give definitive medical care.

Here is how it works:

It is eleven o'clock on a rainy night. The police desk receives a frantic call from Mrs. Schultz. Her husband has just suffered a heart attack and she is all alone with him. Though she is badly frightened she manages to give her address and other relevant information. As soon as she hangs up, the desk clerk repeats to the computer all the facts he has gathered on the Schultz case.

On the basis of current information stored in its memory, the computer immediately selects the type and location of the emergency vehicle best suited to respond to the emergency. An ambulance has just delivered a patient to a hospital and is not very far from the Schultz address. The computer immediately notifies the vehicle crew to proceed to the troubled area. The computer then checks the hospital situation. Before the ambulance has arrived at the Schultz home, the ambulance driver has been notified to take the patient not to the hospital nearby, but to one that has a coronary care unit and is located a few blocks farther away.

Once the ambulance with its patient reaches the hospital the telephone alert takes over. Even while the patient is being carried into the emergency room the nurse in charge picks up the nearest phone and dials a special number. Without waiting for anyone to answer, she says "C-R-T" (for Cardiac Resuscitation Team) and gives the patient's location. The nurse then quickly hangs up and returns to the patient. But all over the hospital the alert goes on. Simultaneously, pocket paging devices carried by physicians begin to buzz, telephones at key locations ring in a way that means emergency—even interrupting calls to get through the recorded message: "C-R-T." Within seconds the Cardiology Department, the Anesthesia Room, the Coronary Care Unit, the on-call rooms, the blood bank, the nurses' station have all been alerted.

At the same time, the emergency cart needed for this particular situation and closest to the patient is automatically turned on to warm up its electronic equipment. In this case of cardiopulmonary arrest, the cart carries an ECG monitor, a resuscitator, defibrillator, oxygen, intravenous equipment, and various drugs and instruments, plus batteries to power the apparatus while it is on its way to the patient.

So that the personnel transporting the cart do not have to lose time waiting for an elevator, an automatic dispatcher sends a car to the floor where the cart is stored. If the patient must be moved, another elevator is sent to that floor. Once the elevator arrives, it locks in place until it is released by a special key.

This whole procedure may sound like something out of a science-fiction movie, but the fact remains that it is saving precious time—and lives—in the hospitals where the project is being tested.

Within two minutes of the first alert, the mobile unit is at the patient's side with a four-person team—an anesthesiologist, a surgical resident, a medical resident, and a nurse. Less than thirty seconds later the emergency cart is being fully utilized. The patient is placed on the litter which is a part of the emergency cart designed by Dr. Nobel and Mr. Rauch. Thus, instead of surrounding the patient with cumbersome equipment, he is fitted into the equipment system and a more efficient man-made relationship results, says Dr. Nobel.

All equipment is stored below the litter's surface. Under the patient's head is a section containing instruments for establishing and maintaining an airway—a respirator, oxygen, suction, and intubation gear. Another section is equipped with a pacemaker, defibrillator, and an ECG direct writer. The cart functions like a miniature coronary cardiac unit.

As the equipment is put to use to reverse the cardiac arrest, a four-channel system records all verbal orders given during resuscitation. Because the emergency nature of resuscitation demands that the physician concentrate exclusively on actions directed toward survival, little thought has been given to research. Dr. Nobel hopes that when enough tapes have been collected, the records will pinpoint errors that have been made and will clearly show the pattern that is most effective for survival.

The emergency system as set up by Dr. Nobel works with equal swiftness whether the problem is a cardiac arrest, a surgical case, or someone seriously injured in an automobile accident.

Recently at Pennsylvania Hospital an eighteen-year-old boy

who had been stabbed in the heart was brought in. He was bled out and cardiac arrest had taken place. He was well on the way to death.

The alert was immediately sounded and within less than a minute the boy was on the litter of the emergency cart. A needle was quickly placed in the sack around the heart to remove the free blood while another doctor started a transfusion in which blood was forced through a vein. Meanwhile, the cardiac compressor was manipulating his heart and the anesthetist was giving him respiration as the cart was moved to the operating theater. Eight minutes after entering the hospital the boy was undergoing emergency surgery. This type of preparation usually takes a minimum of thirty minutes, an interval that is often too long and results in death. In this case, the boy made a good recovery thanks to the quick and expert care he received.

Dr. Nobel and his co-workers hope to have the entire system well documented and ready for use in hospitals throughout the country in a relatively short period of time. The model plan will be applicable to all hospitals whether they are two-elevator, one-hundred-bed institutions in small communities or colossal medical compounds in large cities.

9.
EMERGENCY CARE AROUND THE WORLD

With airplanes flying to the farthermost corners of the earth, automobiles as familiar in Zanzibar as they are in Manhattan, and heavy machinery and mechanical equipment dominating industry, the incidence of accidental deaths has become a major international problem.

In September, 1966, at a meeting in Stockholm, of the International Association and Traffic Medicine, doctors from all over the civilized world assailed the growing toll of injuries and deaths. An international panel of experts declared that a large number of lives could be saved if physicians were better trained to give emergency life-supporting treatment to acutely traumatized patients and if laymen knew such simple procedures as mouth-to-mouth ventilation.

In offering a series of recommendations to all nations, the panel called for expanded medical school training in acute medicine, for complete revision of hospital emergency and ambulance services, and for universal training of the public school population in basic first-aid measures.

"We can no longer be satisfied with first-aid courses concentrating on bandaging, with ambulance services that merely transport the victim, and with emergency rooms not staffed around the clock by physicians experienced in acute medicine," Dr. Peter Safar, who represented the United States on the panel, told the assembly.

Dr. Safar asserted that a major gap in physician education is the lack of training in diagnosing an acute condition in an accident victim and in appropriate methods for giving life-assisting measures. "What is needed is a new specialty, that of resuscitology," he declared.

Dr. Safar believes that if there were universal training of medical men in the definitive care of the injured and if modern resuscitative techniques were taught to the general public, mortality from accidents could be greatly reduced.

Many European countries have organized programs that adequately meet the situation engendered by accidents, sudden death, and other emergencies. For instance, in Austria the victim of an accident is in the hands of well-trained professionals from his first ambulance ride to his last rehabilitation visit to the hospital. These specialists man a unique nationwide system of facilities that are operated by Vienna's General Accident Insurance Company.

The network of trauma facilities includes six accident hospitals, sixteen accident units in general hospitals, and three rehabilitation centers. The entire system is run by the company, which handles the compulsory insurance for Austria's two million workers. Because of the program's success in reducing permanent disability, compensation payments have been reduced and the insurance company, which once operated at a deficit, is now a profitable enterprise.

The patient with serious injuries is rushed by an ambulance that is equipped with medical facilities and manned by trained personnel to a hospital's shock room where a physician specializing in accident surgery and an anesthetist quickly appraise his condition and check his blood pressure, pulse, and reflexes. If necessary he is prepared for surgery on the spot. The hospital has at all times at least one full surgical team on duty no matter what the hour and there are never any delays if surgery is indicated.

At the 250-bed Vienna XII Accident Hospital, there are

twenty-seven full-time doctors; nineteen of them hold a special diploma in accident surgery. This diploma requires at least six years of training, one of which is spent as an anesthetist in an accident hospital.

Directing the Vienna Accident Hospital is senior surgeon Otto Russe, who has thirty years of experience in accident surgery. During 1967, his staff performed fourteen thousand operations.

"Accident surgeons concern themselves with all injuries, no matter where they are located on the body," said Dr. Alfred Wallner, a Kalispell, Montana, surgeon who spent seven months working at the Vienna hospital. "These specialists are so well trained and organized that you could show the same X ray to any one of the fourteen doctors and they would all give you the same diagnosis and prognosis."

But in the whole of the United States there are few trauma centers. One is a twenty-bed unit at Chicago's Cook County Hospital. Accident victims are sent to a general hospital, and the service best equipped to cope with the patient's most serious injury takes over. But Dr. Karl H. Mueller, associate professor of orthopedic surgery at Marquette University, recently pointed out that many accident victims have multiple injuries and need multidiscipline care. To provide such comprehensive care special facilities are needed.

Marquette and Milwaukee County are planning such a project. The proposed accident clinic in Milwaukee will reflect the beginning of a new trend in the United States. Dr. Robert Baker, director of the Chicago trauma facility, notes that at least two dozen hospitals are planning to follow suit.

One of the urgent problems confronting all nations interested in bettering their emergency care is the fact that often patients are lost because of the delay in receiving prompt attention. Transportation to a hospital is basically a communication problem. Belgium, which overcame this problem, instituted a system of emergency telephones at one-mile intervals along the road between Brussels and Ostend. Each of the telephones is tied into a communications network, able to respond by sending an ambulance promptly to the scene of the accident.

In Ireland, cardiologist James F. Pantridge reasoned, as did Dr. Quentin Wood of Southern California, that proper help had to be rushed to the patient, not the patient to the place where he could be properly treated. Too often by the time the patient arrived at the hospital it was too late to help him. Working with other doctors, an ambulance was equipped with all the new and miracle-working equipment that is found in coronary care units.

In the first fifteen months of operation, three hundred victims of heart attacks received intensive care at the place where they were struck down. Not a single patient has been lost.

After the first crisis is over, the patient is carefully moved into an ambulance, and resuscitation—which may include everything from heart massage to electric shock—is continued. At the Royal Victoria Hospital in Belfast the patient is placed in a Coronary Care Unit where he continues to be monitored toward complete recovery.

In Japan, a mobile surgical unit is being tested for emergency use by the Tokai Accident Control Center in Kobe. The automobile-mounted unit consists of a high-pressure oxygen compartment six feet in diameter by ten feet high, fed with purified air and oxygen, and equipped with communication and observation facilities. It can accommodate a doctor and a patient, but three additional patients can be handled if necessary. Health officials believe the unit will be especially useful in bringing quick assistance to victims of traffic or industrial accidents.

In Sweden, Denmark, and Norway, as in Australia, all school children are trained in resuscitative techniques from the age of eight on through high school. The public is urged through radio announcements and newspaper articles to enroll in special classes where they will receive instruction in the handling of emergency situations. Laymen are taught how to recognize unconsciousness, airway obstruction, external bleeding, shock, and pulselessness—and how to treat these conditions. Some advanced classes also teach how to immobilize suspected fractures.

In Stockholm a new course was recently added to the curriculum. Making use of mannequins, laymen are taught how to extricate an unconscious accident victim from auto wreckage.

All experts in emergency care agree that the critically traumatized patient must be brought to a hospital where he can be met and treated by a team of specialists including a general surgeon, neurosurgeon, anesthesiologist, urologist, and orthopedist.

As an example of the kind of institution envisaged, the Hospital Cochin in Paris was cited to doctors who attended the International Congress. The hospital has a traumatologic clinic whose function is to receive the most severe casualties within its district of approximately 600,000 residents. On duty at all times are a general surgeon and a specialist in orthopedic surgery. Available at short notice are a urologist and a neurosurgeon.

The Admissions Department of the Cochin Hospital has fifteen beds, and as a back-up to these there is a large department with 170 beds for orthopedic surgery and burns.

Paris now also has new ambulances available on a twenty-four-hour basis which come equipped with resuscitators and oxygen. An intern is always aboard when the ambulance goes out to pick up an injured person on the highway or an accident victim on the busy city streets. Now authorities in Paris are discussing still another innovation—a helicopter service that will link small hospitals with larger medical centers. The service will transport patients to the hospital or bring a physician to the patient at the accident scene and, after emergency treatment, will take patient and doctor to a hospital where further corrective measures can be taken.

Nor is Paris the only city in France to recognize the problem of emergency care. In Marseilles, there are four hospitals that alternately, approximately every two days, receive all the acute surgery from the entire city.

The Soviet Union has made it mandatory that every doctor —regardless of his specialty—be trained in the use of the newest resuscitation methods. Research on the mechanics of death is a major program, and an essential element of the scientific community is focused on the reversal of unforeseen death.

The Laboratory for Resuscitation of the Organism, where much of the present knowledge of the mechanics of death originated, has been active since 1936. The institute, one of the most famous in the world, is housed in an old four-story building, one of a row of typical Moscow residences. But it has a brilliant staff of research scientists, is equipped with laboratories for physiology, metabolic studies, histology, a soundproof room for conditioned reflexes, and an area for the development of electric equipment.

The institute is headed by Dr. Vladimir Alexandrovich Negovsky, who firmly believes that resuscitation is "one of the most important and urgent medical emergencies."

Dr. Negovsky states: "Resuscitation is a science which is at present only in the early stages of development. Only the crumbs of knowledge have been gathered, only the first stones of the building have been laid. . . ." This is undoubtedly true, but it is also true that the Soviet is far ahead of many other nations in the use they make of the knowledge that is presently available.

In Moscow today there are eighty resuscitation centers. Twenty of them also conduct intensive research. Staffed by specially trained doctors and with the latest equipment always on hand, they go into action without a second's delay. Ambulances manned by expert crews and carrying the necessary equipment answer calls the minute they come in and start resuscitation en route to the nearest station which is rarely more than minutes away.

These stations are not hospitals—they are strictly resuscitation centers where the staff is prepared to immediately administer the emergency measures needed, whether it's electric shock to start the heart, a transfusion, or the giving of oxygen and heart massage to revive a victim of sudden death. Once the patient is over the original crisis, he is sent on to a hospital where he will be given the care he must have for the weeks that follow.

One result of this all-out campaign is that the Soviet Union, which like the United States has a high rate of heart disease, has thousands of victims of fatal coronary attacks leading useful, productive lives. Many of them are alive and active ten and twelve years after being revived from clinical death.

10.
THE MIRACLE OF MOSCOW

One of the most amazing case histories demonstrating what dedicated care can accomplish is that of Dr. Lev Davidovich Landau, acknowledged as the number one scientist of the Soviet Union and recognized as one of the world's outstanding theoretical physicists.

Dr. Landau was in a catastrophic automobile accident that left him so close to death that no doctor held any hope for him. Four times the great scientist went into clinical death. And each time teams of doctors fought death systematically and scientifically. For sixty days he lay in a deep coma—deaf, blind, and speechless, his body completely without reflexes—a coma that many doctors considered irreversible. Not only the life of his body, but the life of his extraordinary brain was in jeopardy.

As a science writer I was deeply interested in the outcome of Dr. Landau's ordeal. When it became obvious that the Soviet Union had drawn an iron curtain around their famous scientist, I flew to Russia to learn for myself what had happened to one of the world's most brilliant minds. This case was to prove a perfect example of what can be accomplished when man sets his heart and mind to preserving a life.

The story of the accident that was to become known as the Miracle of Moscow began on the morning of January 7, 1962, a Sunday of leaden skies, bitter winds, and icy roads. Into this frozen world a Volga sedan ventured out for the eighty-mile trip from Moscow to Dubna, the Soviet Union's research center. Scientist Vladimir Sudakov, owner of the car, was in the driver's seat. By his side was Mrs. Sudakov with a basket of eggs on her lap, a present for friends in Dubna. In the back seat sat Dr. Landau.

Dr. Sudakov drove slowly and carefully for the streets were slick with ice. But as they reached the outskirts of the city, a small girl suddenly ran across the road. Dr. Sudakov swerved to avoid hitting the child. The car went into a spin. Coming from the opposite direction was a heavy truck. The driver tried to brake, but it was impossible on that treacherous highway. The truck skidded and collided with the sedan.

The Sudakovs extricated themselves from the wreckage. They were unhurt. Amazingly, even the eggs were still intact. The truck driver, too, was unscratched. But Dr. Landau, who considered driving unsafe and would ride only as a backseat passenger, took the full force of the crash as the truck plowed into the side of the car. His long legs oddly angled, he lay completely motionless, half in and half out of the car. His chest was caved in, blood flowed from a large gash in his forehead and spurted from his ears.

The truck driver ran to a telephone and dialed Number 3, the first-aid number that can be reached without a coin. He reported the accident, gave the location, and added, "Send an ambulance. One man seems dead."

Within minutes, Landau was on his way to the nearest hospital, Number 50, in Moscow's Timiryazev District.

An attending doctor, bending over him with amazement, cried, "He's still alive!" But Landau was barely breathing and it was clear that he was dying. Later the doctors listed his injuries like a catalogue of doom:

The base of his skull was fractured. There was contusion of the frontal and temporal lobes, and his entire brain was hemorrhaging. Nine ribs were broken. His left lung was punctured and bleeding. His pelvis, pubic, hip, haunch bones, and the head of the left thigh bone were fractured. His bladder was ruptured and the contusions of the abdominal organs were so severe that it was feared other internal organs would rupture. His arms and legs were paralyzed and the vital functions of his body were all but halted. Any one of these injuries could mean death at any moment. Attending physicians administering emergency aid held little hope he would last the day.

When the identity of the injured man became known, the hospital staff urgently started telephoning doctors and scientists throughout the city for aid. Among the first to arrive at the hospital was Peter Kapitsa, Nobel Prize-winning scientist, teacher and friend, who had saved Landau's life when the latter was falsely accused of spying. Now, as Landau lay dying in a small, suburban hospital, Kapitsa, whose status gave him access to anyone at any level, made personal calls to top physcians and sought their help.

Leading surgeons and physicians drafted to care for Landau included orthopedists, blood specialists, nephrologists, nutritionists, urologists, pharmacologists—experts in every medical field. More than one hundred physicians formed the team that worked desperately to keep Landau alive.

Concordia, Landau's beautiful wife, who was among the first notified, drove immediately to the hospital from the country house where she had been staying with their sixteen-year-old son, Igor. Nervous and apprehensive when she arrived, she was unprepared for what awaited her. Her first sight of Landau filled her with such terror that she fainted. Like the doctors who attended him, Concordia did not believe it possible for that broken body ever to mend.

Many of Landau's students and friends who thronged the hospital corridors cried openly as they begged the doctors "to do something." But there was little that could be done. Generally when a badly injured person is brought to a hospital, there is extensive surgery and repair work. But in Landau's case this was out of the question. Any drastic treatment would result in additional trauma and might bring on instant death. The doctors performed stop-gap emergency measures against infection and shock and decided on a "wait-and-see" policy. They would take up each crisis as it arose.

The son of a woman physician and an engineer, Lev Davidovich Landau was born on January 22, 1908, in Baku on the Caspian Sea. A mathematical wizard even as a child, he could hardly remember not being able to solve problems in differential and integral calculus. He entered Baku University at fourteen and received his doctorate five years later from the University of Leningrad.

In that year, 1927, he introduced a concept of energy, called the density matrix, now widely used in quantum mechanics. It was a propitious time for a young genius to make an appearance, for the new Soviet was looking for talent. Lenin recognized that it was the scientists working in their laboratories who were shaping the world of tomorrow. Even as the struggle of the revolution continued, 117 scientific institutions were developed in the Soviet Union.

Two years later Landau was sent abroad for study at scientific centers in Denmark, Switzerland, Germany, and the Netherlands. His stay abroad, working with top scientists, made him one of the world's leading theoreticians. An important influence at this time was Niels Bohr, the renowned Danish physicist, who became Landau's idol as well as his teacher. It was in his years in the West that Dr. Landau began the investigations that led him to the study of low temperature physics.

On his return to the Soviet, Dr. Landau performed the early stages of his research as chief of the theoretical division of the Kharkov Physical and Technical Institute. His intricate theories which helped delineate the world of absolute zero—called cryogenics—won him many awards from admiring Western colleagues. It also brought him a Stalin Prize, a Lenin Prize, the Order of Lenin, as well as the Nobel Prize. Landau's original work opened new scientific vistas and became the subject of intense research in laboratories throughout the world.

While at Kharkov, Dr. Landau met and married Concordia Terentrevna, a chemistry student. A slender, brown-eyed blonde with classic Ukranian features, she was Landau's ideal of feminine beauty.

Dr. Yevgeny M. Lifshitz, who joined Dr. Landau at Kharkov, became his good friend and collaborator. When they moved on in 1937, to Dr. Kapitsa's Institute of Physical Problems in Moscow, they wrote an encyclopedic series of monographs on theoretical physics that has since become a classic.

Apart from his laboratory work, Dr. Landau was a dedicated teacher and popular lecturer with a gift of stating the abstruse in simple terms. He was known never to turn away a student who showed genuine interest in science. His teaching was one of the great contributions that helped place Russia in the ascendency in scientific fields. His school of gifted and devoted pupils was recognized as unique, one that could not be equalled anywhere in the world.

But the political climate in the Soviet Union changed drastically as Stalin consolidated his power. He mistrusted all intelligentsia, especially scientists. Many eminent scientists were jailed, others executed.

In the winter of 1938 Dr. Landau was suddenly arrested on a charge that he was a German spy—a charge that was ridiculous since Landau, a Jew, would hardly be working for Hitler. After a brief interrogation, Landau was sentenced to ten years in prison. For more than a year he languished in a dank, dark cell which he shared with forty other political prisoners. He suffered greatly from the cold and was ill most of the time. He was later to say that he could not have survived another six months.

At this crucial time Peter Kapitsa returned to Moscow. Learning that his protégé was in prison, he immediately arranged to see him. Kapitsa hardly recognized his friend. Landau was frighteningly thin, his hair streaked with gray, his eyes burning with fever.

When Kapitsa learned of the trumped-up charges, he left the prison and drove directly to the Kremlin where he asked to see Vyacheslav Molotov. At the risk of his own life, he laid down an ultimatum—either Landau would be immediately released or he, Kapitsa, would leave the Institute of Physical Problems and refuse to work. That very day Landau was released and driven to the small apartment on the grounds of the institute where his young wife awaited him.

Landau returned to work immediately and fulfilled in great measure the hopes that Kapitsa held for him. The war brought a new urgency to scientific experiments.

His genius continued to flourish long after most scientists have ceased to turn out original research, for science is a young man's field. On his fiftieth birthday, a Soviet article said:

> His inextinguishable enthusiasm for science, his acute criticism, his talent and clarity of thought, attract many young people to "Dau," as his pupils and associates have come to call him.

Until the day of his accident, only two weeks before his fifty-fourth birthday, Landau seemed a man who could laugh at birthdays. Still vigorous and actively producing, he played a leading role in launching the space age.

Now as Landau, unseeing and unhearing, lay in a small suburban hospital, Kapitsa once again took charge of his friend's destiny. Hospital Number 50 was poorly equipped to care for a man as desperately damaged as Landau. But the physicist could not be moved. Even to turn him was dangerous, for doctors feared an embolism—a runaway blood clot forming in an artery that can cause instant death if it hits a vital organ. Because of his drastic internal injuries, his bones remained unset, nor could any major surgery be attempted.

Yet, if he was to survive, he needed expert and dedicated care. Kapitsa set up a rescue headquarters in the hospital. Landau's students, who had gained so much from him, now turned out in force to repay him. A duty roster of volunteers included eighty-nine physicists who were ready and willing to devote their time and strength to saving Landau. Kapitsa organized them into teams—teams which were always on hand to fight death.

Keeping a day-and-night vigil at his bedside, the young physicists, under the supervision of the doctors, undertook the complete medical care of their teacher. They provided him with meticulous minute-by-minute attention, performed the most menial tasks—washed out his stomach, regulated his respiration, doled out medication, sunctioned off mucous and sputum, used syringes to remove blood from the pleura, fed him through tubes.

When problems arose, the scientists came up with ingenious answers. To make it possible to move him, some of the physicists designed a remarkable bed with a special bedspring and inflated mattress that could be adjusted to any position. In this bed he could be turned from one side to the other and his trunk or legs raised separately. When Landau could not breathe for himself, they lugged a respirator from the Moscow Institute of Cardiac Surgery. Those who had cars became chauffeurs, picking up doctors and other personnel at any time of the day or night as they were needed, taking them home when their duties were finished. Others took jobs as messengers, secretaries, porters, supply agents, and menials.

To a large extent, Landau's life was being lived for him. Catheters were premanently implanted in his trachea, his stomach, veins, urinary bladder, and colon. And the artificial breathing apparatus was in continual operation, day and night, for seven weeks. But the onslaught of death persisted from every side. In spite of mass administration of antibiotics to prevent infection of Landau's wounds, infections developed and became virulent. Long an indiscriminate user of antibiotics which he took against colds and other minor ailments which could easily have been treated without them, Landau had built up so strong an immunity that now in his life-and-death struggle they proved ineffective.

Kapitsa alerted Landau's friends throughout the world of the emergency. Hundreds of offers of help came from the scientific communities. In London, Jan Maxwell, who had edited several of Landau's books in English, was particularly touched by the tragedy that had befallen Landau for, only a few days earlier, his own son had been in a similar accident from which he had not yet recovered consciouness. On Maxwell's instructions, a Moscow-bound airliner was detained at the airport to receive a package of special medication. It was labeled simply, "For Mr. Landau." In Copenhagen, Neils Bohr personally arranged for drugs to be sent to his former student and friend. In the next few days, special antibiotics not available in the U.S.S.R. arrived from America, Britain, Belgium, Germany, Czechoslovakia, and Denmark. The "messengers" who picked up the life-saving drugs at the Moscow International and rushed them to the hospital were often world-renowned physicists.

The infections were checked but Landau continued to sink. Medical decisions were often hair-trigger affairs, for even the slightest error could prove fatal. Landau was, from the first, fed through the veins, but self-poisoning set in as a result of the body's inability to control metabolism and elimination of waste products. Prolonged artificial feeding is always dangerous as it results in a disproportion of proteins in the blood, the accumulation of waste products from destroyed cells, and a wavering acid-base balance. The doctors at Landau's side did blood examinations of the fractions of his blood every two or three hours, enabling them to compensate for the missing substances by injection or by mass transfusion of donor blood.

Landau's temperature veered from a high of 107.5° to 104°, a result of the breakdown of cells in the body. Breathing is automatically adjusted to the body's needs—heavier during exercise, deeper and more rapid when fever exhausts the body's oxygen. In Landau's case, the automatic control of oxygen saturation had ceased and had to be carefully regulated by adjusting the respirator with each change in temperature.

But in spite of the medical virtuosity, the new miracle drugs, and the constant care, four days after the accident Landau suddenly succumbed. His pulse disappeared, blood pressure fell to zero, and the EEG—electroencephalograph—tracing flattened out. Clinically, Dr. Landau was dead. But the devoted physicians at his side refused to turn off the respirator.

Instantly the doctors mobilized a giant-killing battle against the irreversible death that was only minutes away. Not even a second could be lost if Landau's magnificent brain was to be saved. While one doctor massaged the heart externally in order to maintain the circulation of the blood, another quickly opened his left radial artery that leads directly to the heart and started a transfusion of fresh blood mixed with strophantin and epinephrine (drugs used to stimulate the heart).

As the transfusion took effect, the manometer immediately showed the rising pressure of blood pushing its way toward the heart. The pump oxygenator was kept working to supply vital oxygen to the brain, while the doctor monitoring the electrocardiograph guided the team of doctors as they fought to reverse the tide of death.

Slowly the heart resumed its beat, the blood pressure rose, and Landau was kept breathing by means of the respirator. But death still hovered close. Three more times—on the seventh, ninth, and eleventh days—Landau went out. Each time clinical death set in, the odds against recovery were greater, yet each time the medical team resuscitated him.

Landau remained barely alive as new and incredible crises arose. He suffered traumatic paralysis of the bowels, ileus, autointoxication, uremia and kidney blockage, traumatic pneumonia, cerebral edema. And his temperature continued to fluctuate.

Always, it seemed, a cure for one ailment created a new

problem in another part of the body. When a swelling of the brain began, the doctors quickly injected urea to counteract it. Immediately an excess of the urea blocked the kidneys, which were no longer able to eliminate the body's waste products. Uremia, the dangerous accumulation in the blood of residual nitrogen compounds, set in. A new group of specialists gathered around Landau's bed. The urologists came up with an effective treatment and slowly the kidneys returned to their normal function.

The persistent irritation from injuries and infection plus the immobility of the body in prone position on its back brought on hypostatic pneumonia—a general inflammation of the lungs.

The use of the new antibiotic drugs flown in from the West and the devoted care overcame the pneumonia, vanquished the high fever. Five weeks after the accident the fractures had ossified. Infections had disappeared. Both lungs were healed and functioning normally in spite of the frightful injuries they had received. As those improvements took place, Landau's digestion benefited and it was possible to put him on a regular diet, to discontinue intravenous feeding, and to introduce food directly into the stomach through a thin plastic tube in the nose.

The Soviet's chief dieticians, who conferred with the medical team, dreamed up menus that were not only nutritious but of gourmet quality. Many of the foods came from foreign lands. Fresh oranges, grapefruits, and dates imported from Egypt; grapes grown in the hothouses of the Crimea; fresh fish and the best caviar from the Black Sea; crabs from the Baltic—all were flown in daily. These carefully selected foods so rarely seen in Moscow during the long winter months were measured, crushed, and reduced to a uniform paste sufficiently liquid to be poured down a tube. For the comatose Landau, the new diet made little difference because he had neither taste nor appetite. But the fresh, vitamin-rich foods accomplished their purpose. They brought new life to the body of the emaciated physicist.

Though Landau's battered body survived and, indeed, had

begun to show signs of recovery, he still remained totally unconscious, his extremities completely paralyzed. He had no pain reaction, and neither flashes of light near his eyes nor rattling at
his ears brought any response. Landau did not even have breathing reflexes at this time. If the respirator was disconnected, his
chest would rise and fall for a few seconds, then come to a complete stop—a sign that no part of his brain was functioning.

The doctors were plagued by fear. Would their heroic
fight for Landau's life end in disaster? Never had they worked
on a case like this, for never had a patient who suffered such
massive injuries recovered to live normally. The question that
tormented Landau's physicians was: Could Landau's brilliant
mind be saved or—if he survived—would he continue to live on as
a vegetable, a mindless body?

Whether a doctor should preserve a life that would prove a
burden and a tragedy often has been debated by the medical
profession. Even as the Soviet doctors battled for Landau's life,
a great medical controversy raged. Some doctors spoke out
against the desperate measures to keep the scientist alive. What
was the point, they asked, if he would live on as an idiot? By
implication, *Lancet*, Britain's noted medical journal, concurred
when it editorialized that doctors should not seek to prolong the
lives of brain-damaged patients who lay in an "irrevocable
coma." By accepted medical standards, Landau, who remained
unconscious for sixty days, was in such a coma.

Kapitsa, who had masterminded much of Landau's care,
now proposed that they seek help from the West and hold an
international consultation. Landau's physicians, the very finest in
all of Russia, agreed.

Seven weeks after the accident, Soviet doctors asked for
help from the free world. Dr. Wilder Penfield, Canada's famed
neurosurgeon, flew from Montreal at a few hours' notice. Drs.
Gerard Guillot and Marie Garcin of France and Dr. Sdenck
Kunz of Czechoslovakia came to Moscow for the conference.
They were not hopeful. Dr. Kunz voiced the belief of all of

them when he stated: "The traumas sustained are incompatible with life."

The doctors argued among themselves, for they could not agree on the extent of the brain injuries. The urgent question was whether there was one large hematoma—blood clot—pressing upon neighboring tissues and arteries and destroying more cells around it or numerous small hemorrhages. A large hematoma should be removed surgically, as it could totally destroy the brain by pressing on neighboring tissues and squeezing capillary arteries, thereby depriving them of oxygen. But if the injury consisted of small hemorrhages, they might better be left alone, in the hope they would heal themselves in time.

The question resolved itself when Dr. Penfield, reexamining the patient, detected the first glimmer of consciousness. "His eyes seemed to focus on me," Dr. Penfield said. "I moved my head. They followed. His eyes were the only part of his body not completely paralyzed."

Dr. Penfield advised against a brain operation. Before leaving Moscow, he had Landau moved to the Institute of Neurosurgery and outlined a complete program of rehabilitation and therapy.

The electroencephalographs (the graphic record of the brain's activity) which were used throughout the illness in an effort to estimate the brain damage, showed an abnormal rhythm at this time. But four months after the accident, the pattern was normal and the impulses began going through the machine.

This was encouraging, for the doctors believed that the return of some cerebral function indicated that the damage to the brain consisted chiefly in this disconnection between the cells which could be repaired in time. But a real understanding of neurophysiological processes, the most fundamental notions about brain functions, are still lacking. The doctors could not be sure that further improvement would take place.

Then, suddenly, Landau began to talk. His speech was halting, sometimes garbled. As the days passed, he learned to speak

134

Four Minutes to Life

as a child does, by repeating words and phrases that were spoken to him.

The early memories of his childhood and student days were the first to return. This is the usual pattern, for in childhood and youth the brain is less specific, less economical than in a grown man. It has not been trained yet, and a larger portion of the cortex is taken up by the recording of the first memories. Later, regions of the brain become specialized for different types of thought processes, and memories seem to become restricted to more specific areas.

From the beginning, Landau's mind, with its amazing capacity for imaginative abstraction and reasoned recollection, created its own patterns. The restoration of his higher psychic functions progressed in a complex, torturous way.

At this time he could not recall the most basic facts of his life. Yet when a friend started reciting a verse from Pushkin's poem, "Eugene Onegin," it instantly came back to him and he was able to continue without faltering.

Landau's mind seemed to fade in and out. When a doctor addressed him in French, he automatically answered in French, though his speech remained halting. But when a nurse pointed to a ring on her finger and asked, "What is this?" his brow furrowed in deep concentration.

Finally he answered: "A watch."

His speech became clearer day by day. From the beginning, Landau was impatient to get back to a normal life. Long before he was out of bed, he had made it clear that he hated and was bored with hospital routine. When his friends visited him, he wanted to talk shop, to be a part of their world.

One evening his friend Lifshitz asked Landau to solve a complicated problem. Landau thought a moment or two and gave an answer. He then closed his eyes. A physician who was standing nearby looked questioningly at Lifshitz, who sadly shook his head. "It's wrong," he whispered. Later, however, when he mulled over the problem, Lifshitz suddenly realized that Landau's solution was correct. Landau had simply arrived at the answer through a new route, an approach that had not even occurred to Lifshitz. Landau's mind was apparently using new pathways.

His recovery continued at an erratic pace. Someone would mention an incident from his past and he would smile, yet at times he could not remember the names of even his best friends. There were days when his progress seemed remarkable, but at other times it bogged down. No one could predict with certainty whether he would ever fully recover his exceptional reasoning power or whether he would even be able to take his place in a normal society.

Landau's physical condition improved, but he was still suffering from a strong, nagging pain in his left leg. Attempts to treat the pain with massage and heat or with other classical means failed. Nor did it respond even temporarily to massive injections of novocain. Week after week, month after month, the pain persisted. Nothing seemed to help. Doctors treating him felt that there was no doubt the pain resulted from damage to the brain, probably affecting a small region, perhaps only a few cells, in the thalamus, the mass of gray nerve matter at the base of the brain.

A standard method of treatment of such an injury would have been to irradiate the appropriate area with X rays. But in Landau's case they did not dare—they could not assume the risk of adding further injury to the brain, to use a treatment that might prevent complete medical recovery later.

Psychologists say that there is nothing so debilitating as uninterrupted pain. As it continued, Landau became weary and discouraged. When old friends visited him, his courtesy and love of people asserted itself. At such times he roused himself and made an effort to be warm and friendly. But these efforts were sporadic. Aware of his circumstances, his memory lapses caused him great anguish and forced him to withdraw more and more.

A hospital is a world apart and Landau had become part of

it—the outside world and its interests seemed far away. Day by day the slow monotony of the hospital routine ate more deeply into him. He no longer struggled against it, no longer talked of leaving, of going back to work. Step by step he had been driven into an isolation and loneliness of the soul.

His doctors were baffled. Had he made as much progress as he could? The physicians and psychiatrists who were trying to help Landau found that often they were treading on the thin air of inadequate fundamental knowledge. For what is the mechanism of memory, the anatomy of intelligence? How can these intangible facilities be related to the shape, the size, the particular manner in which some sixteen billions of nerve cells are assembled in the brain? There is no clear definition. As scientists study the intricacies of the mind, perform experiments on animals and on humans, their concepts are constantly changing.

Landau's physicians and the neurological specialists who treated him gathered many times to review the most recent basic knowledge on memory and brain function—knowledge that was rapidly expanding even as Landau lay in the hospital. In the last decade, there has been an increasing amount of evidence to indicate that memory is stored chemically, as an accumulation of structural, biochemical alterations, spread through a large number of cells and in many regions of the brain. It is now known that ribonucleic acid (RNA) plays an important role in the memory processes of higher forms of life. The nervous impulses coming to the brain, it seems, stimulate, and transform molecules of RNA as if imprinting upon them a coded message that becomes memory.

In experiments, patients who received injections of RNA showed a marked improvement in their ability to remember in comparison to those who received none. The doctors caring for Landau considered the possibility of RNA injections but rejected the idea, for at that time, treatment with RNA could cause unpleasant side effects, particularly dangerous in patients whose physical condition was already poor or fragile. (More recent experiments have taken most of the bugs out of the chemical. A new drug, Cylert, which has been given long and exhaustive tests, holds a definite promise that in the near future memory can be restored by its use.)

When the international "brain trust" left Moscow, Landau disappeared from the news. But on November 1, he was again on the front pages of the world's newspapers when the Nobel Committee in Stockholm announced that Lev Davidovich Landau had been awarded the 1962 Nobel Physics Prize for original research on theories regarding the fluidity of helium at low temperatures, a field in which he pioneered.

Friends and colleagues everywhere felt Landau richly deserved the prize. The fact that he was still very ill added a poignant note. Had Landau been well, the news would have been received in his lecture hall amidst the tumult of his students, the congratulations of his friends. And, after thirty years, there would have been the keen delight of preparing for a trip to the outside world. This was only the fourth time that the Nobel Prize for Physics had gone to the Soviet Union, and there was no doubt Landau would have been permitted to attend the ceremonies in Stockholm.

Instead, on December 10, 1962, the presentation took place in the environs of the small hospital where Landau had known so many tortured hours. It was the first time, except in wartime, that the award was made outside of Sweden.

It was a sad ceremony. Though it was arranged at the same time that the Laureates would be receiving their awards from King Gustav VI there was little similarity between the two events. Landau, very frail, was propped up in a chair. A group of doctors stood by as Swedish Ambassador Rolf R. Sohlman congratulated the scientist in the name of the Royal Academy and the King of Sweden. The presentation ceremony was over in a few minutes and the ambassador found himself outside; he had not been permitted to talk to Landau.

After the story of the award, a reign of silence descended

about Landau, his progress, and his activities. Except for an occasional announcement issued by the Soviet Academy of Science
to the effect that Landau was "making progress," there was no
news. Visiting scientists, friends of Landau, were told he was
unable to receive visitors. No reporter was permitted to interview him.

But Landau's condition continued to raise conjectures. According to some authorities, he was making a full recovery, both
physically and mentally. Others insisted that Landau was no
longer the man who had been recognized as one of the great
minds of the twentieth century—that the desperate measures for
his recovery had been in vain.

Was the saving of Landau's life really the triumph for
science that the Russians claimed? Was he making a complete recovery and thereby reversing medical history, or had the brilliant mind of one of the world's leading scientists been tragically
lost?

As a science reporter, I had kept up with the Landau case
from the beginning. Now that the news had abruptly stopped, I
wondered what the true situation was.

At a convention of the American Medical Association, I
spoke to a number of brain specialists about Landau. Not one
of them believed it possible for the scientist to make a satisfac-
tory recovery from his extensive brain injuries.

But one doctor told me: "Since World War I, there have
been great advances in the knowledge of the brain. But the end
results of the survivor of brain damage are always uncertain.
There are often deep changes in personality." The doctor
thought a moment, then resumed softly, as if talking to himself: "I have a case now—a little girl who was in a bad accident. We operated on her brain. When she came to, she seemed
to be an idiot. But after two months she began to come back.
She's almost normal now. There's still a lot we don't know. . . ."

When I had an opportunity to go to Russia, I decided to

try to find out for myself how Landau was faring. The Soviet Cultural attaché stationed in Washington, D.C., told me it would be impossible to set up an interview with Dr. Landau from New York. I was advised to get in touch with the Academy of Sciences in Moscow.

Six weeks later, I received an answer from the academy. It could not grant an interview. Dr. Landau was still ill.

But it had been almost two years since the accident; surely he was able to see people. I flew to Russia. Very quickly, I ran into the Russian "Nyet!" Since an official interview would have to be set up through the academy, I went there first. I explained I was a science writer visiting the Soviet Union. The discussion went smoothly until I mentioned Landau. Suddenly the veneer of politeness vanished and the director was shouting. "You will not see Landau! No one will see him!"

"But why?" I asked, incredulous at the sight of the official, red in the face and yelling at the top of his voice.

"Only Americans would ask for an appointment. They stop at nothing!" He remembered my letter and looked at me accusingly. "We wrote you not to come."

"I'm a reporter. I have a right to pursue my job," I defended myself.

He calmed down. "Why don't you see something of Moscow? Now that you are here, you might as well enjoy yourself."

As I left the academy, I kept wondering why they were so unwilling for anyone to see Landau. Were they shielding him, conserving his strength? Were they planning a spectacular public appearance when he was fully recovered? Or was it true that Landau was merely a shell, a symbol of what he had once represented?

One thing was clear—I was not going to receive official sanction for the interview. It was months since the last stereotyped release on Landau had been issued by the academy. Landau's address was not listed in the telephone directory, nor was it given in *Who's Who*, and it was possible he was not in Moscow at all. I could find no one who had seen him since his illness. Most of the correspondents in the Moscow press corps considered my task hopeless. Some thought Landau was dead, while others were certain he was hidden away and that no foreigner would ever see him again.

I kept on seeking new contacts, knocking on new doors, and I continued to run into stone walls and impediments, such as Marguerite, a trim young redhead who appeared my first morning in Moscow and announced she was my official Intourist guide. After that she arrived every day as I was having breakfast and stayed glued to my side all day. She insisted I do the tourist bit. "You haven't seen Lenin's Tomb or the Pushkin Museum," she'd remind me. Day after day, she hauled me around the city's shrines and museums and was instantly suspicious if I so much as demurred.

When I complained to one of the correspondents that Marguerite treated me as if I were Mata Hari, he answered quite seriously, "As far as the U.S.S.R. is concerned, you might as well be Mata Hari. In their eyes, you are a spy. Your room is probably wired, your phone tapped, and your every movement reported on. But don't worry about it. It's a way of life."

Every day after Marguerite left, I resumed my search. Just as I was growing discouraged, a door opened. I cannot reveal how I got my information; it would endanger others. But I was introduced to a person who knew Landau and was willing to help me. From him, I learned that Dr. Landau was now a patient at the Academy of Sciences Hospital, a little-known institution used only for scientists. Most important, I learned that he took therapeutic walks in the hospital garden twice daily—in the morning and again in the evening.

Very early next morning—before my guide arrived—my friend drove me to the hospital. Without him, it would have been impossible to find my way, for, though the address is listed as Leninsky Prospect, the hospital is hidden and it is only by cutting off into a short, dead-end street that you arrive at the entrance.

A forbidding wall surrounded the grounds. Large signs stated that anyone entering would be subject to arrest. Trying to look as if we belonged there, we walked in. The place appeared almost empty. We found a bench in a secluded corner and waited.

The hospital, a small, squat building, dominated the grounds, known euphemistically as "the gardens." They were untidy and poorly kept. There was not even one flower bed.

An hour passed. Occasionally a passerby glanced at us, then walked on. The tension had grown almost unbearable, when the front door of the hospital opened for a tall, cadaverous figure wearing hospital pajamas and a warm coat. Leaning heavily on his canes and supported by a nurse, he slowly made his way down the walk. It was Landau.

We watched his painful progress for a few minutes, then moved toward him. Signs of his near-fatal illness were clearly visible. His once dark hair was almost all white, the fine, clear skin looked transparent, and the dark, penetrating eyes were deeply shadowed. On closer observation, a slight droop to his left eyelid was noticeable.

My companion greeted the doctor, then introduced me. To my delight, Dr. Landau acknowledged the introduction in English. I asked him if he would grant me an interview.

"I'm sorry, not now," he said after a moment's hesitation. "I have just had a treatment and I am in much pain." Though the morning was chilly, his forehead was beaded with perspiration and his hands were shaking. I moved back, recognizing the enormity of all this man had suffered and was still suffering. I started to apologize for intruding but he quickly put me at ease.

"It's all right. Perhaps you will be able to come back later when I am feeling better." I had the feeling that the pain was so intense he could hardly stand, but his courtesy and gentleness were instinctive.

As I walked away, I remembered a scientist telling me that Landau was famous for his original scientific research but loved for his wonderful personality—that he was very different from the stereotyped picture of a scientist. Warm and friendly, with an outgoing, generous nature, he was the sort of person who called forth an intensely personal response from people everywhere. More than ever, I wanted a chance to talk to him. His pain, I was told, was acute during the early part of the day. He had asked me to come back. I decided to try again. My problem was getting to the hospital. I couldn't ask my original contact to take the risk a second time. And I was afraid to take a taxi. The driver might turn me in.

Three days later, having nervously waited all day for my guide to leave, I called a man who had helped me on other occasions and asked him to drive me to the hospital. He was fearful but finally consented.

It was after six when I slipped through the forbidden gate. There were people about, but they seemed engrossed in themselves. On a bench at the far left, Landau was sitting quietly, watched over by his nurse, the lonely sadness of his expression reflecting his surroundings.

A lovely smile illuminated his face, highlighting its spiritual beauty as he made room for me on the bench. For fifteen minutes, we talked—the first interview Landau had granted since his accident. The nurse, a plump, matronly woman who spoke no English, was holding his hand all the while.

He seemed to welcome the intrusion, the chance to talk, to forget his surroundings. Free of intense pain and relaxed, he was enjoying himself. There was still about him the eagerness and the warmth that made him "Dau" to all his friends. It was easy to see in him the man whose wit and charm could keep any company in a state of hilarity.

Landau's English was fluent and without accent. When I commented, he said, "Yes, it was not difficult for me to learn languages again. [He spoke English, French, and German.] And everything I ever knew about physics came back, too. But I remember nothing of the accident. It's still a blank."

Apparently, it had happened too quickly and it still seemed

inexplicable. His only real memory was of the fearful awakening to a world in which everything he knew, everything he valued, seemed to have been swept away by one terrible stroke of fate.

He recalled that when he awoke to a nightmare world, he had no idea where he was or who he was. His first reaction on recovering consciousness was, "What am I doing here?"

He laughed wryly as he told me, "I didn't even know my own wife. I accused her of being an imposter. When she tried to reason with me, I insisted she was a murderess, that she had killed my real wife and kidnapped my son."

"I've seen her picture," I said. "She's very beautiful."

"She's much more than just beautiful." Landau's voice was warm with pride. "She is very clever. And so patient. Without her, it would have been much more difficult."

Landau told me that when he first recovered consciousness after his sixty-day coma, he started living through the stages of his life all over again, beginning with his infancy, and passing on through childhood until he was again an adult. He had to learn to breathe, to speak, to hear, to walk. To master the most simple skills took hours of practice.

But Landau didn't want to dwell on hospitals, medications, therapy. He obviously found the role of invalid an unhappy and frustrating one. It seemed to me that he lived on two planes— one in which his pain-racked body submitted to the ministrations of doctors and nurses, and another where his brilliant, restless mind escaped into spheres of its own.

As his health improved, he began to take an increasing interest in the outside world, resumed some family responsibilities. Possibly because of the emotional upheaval engendered by the accident, his son, Igor, came close to failing in his school studies. Mrs. Landau was worried.

"He's not working, enough," she confided to her husband. "I'm afraid he's going to fail his university entrance exams."

Dr. Landau set about rectifying the situation. He worked

out a series of tests that he gave to Igor over a period of weeks. He was back in his own sphere and could reassure his wife: "Don't worry. I'm sure he'll make it." And Igor did.

Except for the black-out on the accident, which doctors felt was partly psychological, Landau's mind and memory seemed to be fully restored. I had heard there were plans for him to return to the university to teach.

"Yes, I hope to teach again," Dr. Landau confirmed. For a moment his face looked alive and happy.

But at my next question—"When do you think you'll be able to start?"—a shadow passed over his face and his voice lost its vibrancy. Like most people who have endured severe illness, he alternated between hope and despair, was fearful that his travail would never end.

"I have been in the hospital almost two years. Who can tell when I'll teach again. . . ." The defenselessness of the sick was in his voice. Landau, who could spend long cycles of time buried in his laboratory and emerge with a zest, a love of life, a feeling of accomplishment, now viewed time at the other end of the telescope. He would soon be fifty-six and time seemed to be flying by.

While in the hospital, he worked out a series of new theories for teaching physics to the young. But the long, dreary months had made him doubt their value, as well as his ability to regain his place in life. A deep bitterness broke through his gallantry.

"There is so much for me to catch up—so much has happened in physics." His face was desolate as he added mockingly, "Perhaps all I'm good for is to sit on a bench. I'm a broken thing."

It had grown colder and there was rain in the air. I felt I was tiring him and rose to go. With almost visible effort, he pushed aside his despondency.

"Come and see me again," he urged cordially.

It was obvious Dr. Landau had no idea of the strict vigil that kept him secluded, that his very existence was shrouded in secrecy.

I could not forget the heartbreak in his voice toward the end of the interview. Was he right when he said, "All I'm good for is to sit on a bench"?

I decided to interview some of the doctors who had seen Landau through his long illness. In Moscow, I saw Dr. Vladimir Alexandrovich Negovsky, who is responsible for much of the present knowledge of the mechanics of death.

A large, graying man, world-famous for his original techniques, Dr. Negovsky spoke of Landau's recovery as a "miracle." Negovsky does not use the word "miracle" lightly. He was not referring to the fact that Landau had been resuscitated, for he does not look upon resuscitation from clinical death as sorcery but as a medical fact, to which every man is entitled. The miracle was that he was alive at all, for Landau's injuries were so grave that no doctor in the world looking at him those first weeks after the accident would have given him one chance in a hundred for survival.

Dr. Negovsky made it clear that the fact that Landau lived was a result of the years of intense research that went into developing modern methods of resuscitation. Had Landau's accident occurred in the early fifties, he would not have recovered.

Dr. Negovsky stated that Landau's recovery was complete. "His intellect and ability to think deeply and logically have been restored. He is making remarkable progress—he does not realize himself how far he has come. He will be as well as ever when he leaves the hospital."

Dr. Michael Grashchenkov, who had been with Landau through the entirety of his long illness, said of him: "He would be considered cured—if he weren't Landau. But as one of the world's top physicists, he will not be entirely cured until he starts working again."

On February 2, 1964, three months after I interviewed Landau, the Moscow radio announced that he had been released from the hospital.

Landau was still suffering pain, but his doctors had realized that he was sinking into a condition known as "hospital syndrome," a general apathy, an indifference that threatens to over-come any patient who remains bedridden too long. The results of a physical checkup by Dr. Grashchenkov appeared at this time in *Medical World News*: Landau's torn lung had com-pletely healed, his breathing was normal, and his heart was in excellent shape. Because none of the classic methods of treating fractures could be used while he was ill, Landau's left leg was two centimeters shorter than the right. "Throughout his long illness, doctors have had difficulty in subduing the pain in his leg, as it does not react to procaine or other pain killers," Dr. Grashchenkov stated, adding that the pain was gradually disap-pearing.

Dr. Grashchenkov said of Landau's psychological health: "He has shown amazing courage, remarkable persistence and stamina. The long travail is bound to affect him at times. But Landau will recover completely."

Landau began to show marked improvement as soon as he got out of the hospital. The apartment in which he had lived for so many years and from which he had walked out one bitter cold morning two years earlier, had been readied for him. The stair-case leading to the second floor had been widened, a new bath-room built next to his room, and steel handles attached to the walls, the bannister, and even to his bed, to enable him to grasp one handle, then another as he walked along, haltingly but with-out crutches.

Back in his own environment, Landau's zest for living, his deep interest in science returned full force. He still suffered from pain but it no longer was as severe, and at times it com-pletely disappeared.

As soon as the weather turned warm, he accompanied his family to his country home where his general health was much better and his walking improved. As his health benefited and spirits rose, the pain would disappear sometimes for hours at a time.

Freed of the monster that had imprisoned him for so long

a time, Landau returned to his old vocations. He read voraciously the scientific books, periodicals, and papers that had appeared during his illness. He wrote a long article which was printed in the *Komsomolskaya Pravda* on July 8, 1964, on the occasion of the seventieth birthday of his friend Peter Kapitsa. Much of the article was devoted to Kapitsa's accomplishments as an eminent scientist, but it did not forget the man who as Landau's friend had shown great kindness, honesty, and great humanity.

During the summer, Landau continued to coach his son, Igor, who was studying physics at Moscow University, and the relationship between father and son deepened.

On a sparkling day in October, 1965, Landau once again faced his students at the Moscow Institute for Experimental Physics. His face unlined and tanned, he looked young, healthy, and vital as he addressed his class. His students were aware that his criticisms were as sharp and accurate as before the accident.

It is the old Landau, friends said. His personality had fully returned. Once more he was outgoing, gay, and brilliant. But the long travail was not forgotten. His health was still poor, for he never completely recovered from the terrible injuries inflicted during the accident. But now that he was at home, he made a valiant effort to resume the life he had known. His laughter and high spirits were a protective screen. For the long, terrible illness, the excruciating pain which still returned intermittently, and the tortuous way back had left scars, both physical and psychological. Each morning as he pulled himself up by the rail at the side of his bed, as he walked with painful slowness, he was reminded anew that his body was no longer whole.

As he read books and papers on physics published during the years of his illness, he again realized how much he had missed. But having been so close to death, having faced utter dissolution, life was more meaningful than ever before. He was deeply grateful for the years that had been granted him. To a friend he said: "I am not fully recovered. But I can walk, I can

talk to friends. I can read. Sometimes violent pains attack me.
I can't resist them, not because they are beyond human tolerance
but because I am afraid of them."

But in spite of the pain and illness he continued to teach and
even attempted some research, which was the great love of his
life.

Dr. Landau lived four years after he left the hospital. On
April 1, 1968, the brilliant and beloved scientist met his fifth and
final death.

In a typical tribute at the time of his death, Dr. Hanz Bethe
of Cornell University, who is also a Nobel Prize physicist, ex-
tolled Dr. Landau as "one of the greatest theoretical physicists
of our time." And Dr. Gerog Uhlenbeck of Rockefeller University stated: "Physicists are not yet born who have the same wide
grasp of the science."

Dr. Landau, who acted as a trail blazer in his chosen field
of science, whose original research opened many doors, was able
even in his darkest hour of pain and illness to set a precedent
that will benefit mankind. For to doctors, everywhere, Landau's
recovery, his ability to resume his work, was more than a dramatic and courageous episode. In his successful fight for life and
the life of his mind, the great scientist made medical history. No
longer is it possible to say: "Better not to save a person who has
suffered brain injury." Dr. Landau proved that the inevitable
can be reversed.

11.
HOW TO USE RESUSCITATIVE TECHNIQUES

Our modern resuscitative techniques which are so effective in restoring life were known to man two thousand years ago, and perhaps even before that. Mouth-to-mouth breathing is reported on in the Bible. In Genesis, Chapter 2, Verse 7, we are told the Lord God breathed into Adam's nostrils the breath of life, and Man became a living soul. The Second Book of Kings, Chapter 4, Verse 34, tells of the prophet Elisha who put his mouth upon the mouth of the dead Shunamite child; the child sneezed seven times and opened his eyes.

And there are documents establishing the fact that more than a hundred years ago a young doctor used mouth-to-mouth breathing and closed-heart massage when Abraham Lincoln was fatally wounded while attending the theater on the night of April 4, 1865. The use of these techniques instituted by twenty-three-year-old Dr. Charles A. Leale prevented instant death. Lincoln's life was prolonged for nine hours—a crucial time that averted a nationwide panic. When Lincoln died the next morning, another President had taken over and the continuity of the republic was confirmed.

Today these techniques are still performing miracles. But now we know that the remarkable results that so often turn back death and assure a second chance at life are based on scientific principles.

It was during World War II that medical men began concentrating their efforts on perfecting new and daring resuscitative techniques. Open-heart massage—a drastic procedure that required the slashing open of the chest and could be undertaken only by a doctor—preferably a surgeon—came into wide use. This routine saved thousands of lives in the operating rooms and hospitals. But for the tens of thousands who died suddenly in their homes, while at work, on the golf course, or driving a car little could be done.

Intensive research by three Johns Hopkins Hospital investigators on resuscitative methods culminated in 1960 in the development of the effective cardiopulmonary resuscitative system which today is used throughout the civilized world. For the first time resuscitation that could reverse death became applicable to the public. Many laymen who have become familiar with the medical counterplot for death have used it effectively in life-and-death emergencies.

"The tragedy is that for every life we save by these techniques, probably a dozen are lost because mouth-to-mouth resuscitation and closed-heart massage are not used," says Dr. James R. Jude, past chairman of the American Heart Association's Committee on Emergency Cardiac Pulmonary Resuscitation. He points out that too few people in this country have received training in the modern methods of returning life to the victims of sudden death. Yet tests show that these skills, which even a child can learn, could save more than 100,000 people every year, when properly used.

To perform these life-saving techniques requires no instruments or gadgets. With their two hands and the breath in their lungs, any man, woman, or teen-ager can give a second chance to the heart that has stopped beating. Today anyone can save a life. The new knowledge available cloaks all of us with a new responsibility if death deposits a victim at our feet. What we do in the first minute or two can literally mean the difference between life and death.

No matter what the cause of clinical death—whether the result of accident or heart attack—the initial treatment is always the same. Emergency cardiopulmonary resuscitation involves the following steps:

A. OPEN THE AIRWAY. Provide the patient with an unobstructed airway by hyperextending the head and by clearing the mouth and throat of foreign material.

B. RESTORE BREATHING. Ventilate the patient via mouth-to-mouth or mouth-to-nose breathing until a doctor takes over or respiration returns.

C. RESTORE CIRCULATION. The heart should be compressed manually by techniques used for external cardiac compression.

If the victim is unconscious, the airway must be opened immediately. Often this alone will allow the victim to breathe. During normal breathing air flows easily through the nose or mouth to and from the lungs. But when a person loses consciousness the head tends to slump forward and the relaxed tongue can completely block the movement of air through his throat. Opening the air passage may bring returned consciousness.

The simplest way to keep the tongue from blocking the airway is to *place one hand under the neck and lift. Tilt head back as far as possible by holding the crown of the head with your other hand*. This opens the mouth and removes the tongue from the throat. This operation should be done rapidly—taking no more than a few seconds.

Then, if the victim is not breathing or his breathing efforts are feeble, START RESCUE BREATHING IMMEDIATELY. If practical, place the victim on his back or halfway on his side. However, rescue breathing can be done with the victim sitting in an automobile, pinned under debris, suspended on a safety belt, on an electric power line, or floating face up in the water—as long as you have access to his nose and mouth.

Don't waste time by moving the victim, waiting till a doctor arrives, calling the police, firemen, or members of the family. *Get someone else to do it* while you keep death at bay. Remember that only a short time without oxygen can cause serious damage to the brain. The sooner the circulation is started the better the likelihood of success.

The first blowing effort will determine whether or not obstruction exists. If there is no movement of the chest, quickly check to see if the tongue is blocking the air passage. If something is stuck in the windpipe or throat of an adult victim, place him on his side and apply a sharp blow to his back between his shoulder blades. Hold his mouth open and sweep your fingers through his throat and remove material that is visible. But do it only if you can do it very fast. *Remember that the urgent need is to get air into the lungs even if it has to be blown past whatever is lodged in the throat.* As long as rescue breathing continues, an adult can be kept alive even though his air passage is blocked by a piece of meat or other obstructing material.

After you have inflated the lungs rapidly three to five times, determine if the heart is beating. Maintain backward tilt of the head while feeling for the victim's carotid (neck) pulse with the other hand. The carotid arteries, which are normally large and exhibit strong pulses, lie in the neck on both sides of the windpipe. Feel the pulse only on one side. Do it quickly so as not to interrupt resuscitation. Place two fingers on the Adam's apple and slide them off to the side. Then press gently backward on the neck. If you do it correctly, the carotid artery should lie under your two fingers. Do not cross over the neck with your fingers in order to feel the pulse on the opposite side, since this may obstruct the airway.

If the carotid pulse is strong, continue ventilation, giving twelve to sixteen lung inflations per minute. But if the pulse is absent, *start closed-chest massage without delay.* (This will be explained in detail later.) Even if the diagnosis of cardiac arrest is not quite certain, begin closed-heart massage, for the faint heart action will not supply enough circulation to keep the brain alive. Avoid delay. Every second counts. Properly applied resuscitation is harmless while delay can be fatal.

Successful resuscitation, which requires both mouth-to-mouth breathing and closed-heart massage, ideally should be undertaken by a two-person rescue team. But if you work alone at first, proceed with external cardiac compression after you have ventilated the lungs rapidly from three to five times. After each fifteen compressions ventilate the lungs rapidly two or three times, taking no more than five seconds to do so. Repeat the cycle while yelling for help. If no one is in the house, knock the telephone receiver off the hook, and dial the operator for help.

As soon as help is available, let someone take over the mouth-to-mouth breathing while you continue compressing the heart strongly sixty to eighty times a minute. Your partner will be doing mouth-to-mouth breathing at the rate of twelve to sixteen times a minute. Ideally, inflations should be spaced between every fifth and sixth compression. The compressions should be rhythmic and regulated. It is important to remember that in cases of circulatory standstill, *neither artificial ventilation nor artificial circulation alone is useful.*

The effectiveness of the compression should be checked frequently by someone other than the person applying the pressure. Proof of effectiveness is a good carotid pulse that can be felt after each compression. Other favorable evidence is the constriction of dilated pupils, occasional gasping respiration, purposeful movement of the body, and improved color of the skin.

Even if the patient seems not to be responding, never stop resuscitative efforts until he has arrived at a hospital and doctors have taken an electrocardiogram; resuscitation is incomplete without it. The patient may be suffering from ventricular fibrillation—irregular, spastic contractions resulting in the total loss of heart sounds. The condition is impossible to distinguish from cardiac arrest even with a stethoscope. The use of a defibrillater often shocks the heart back to a normal beat.

While continuing treatment, the rescuer must get someone to summon an ambulance and/or a physician. The person who initiates emergency heart-lung resuscitation has two responsibilities: first, to apply emergency measures to prevent irreversible change to the vital centers of the body; and second, to be sure the victim gets to definitive medical care including hospitalization.

RESCUE BREATHING FOR ADULT VICTIMS

The following procedures should be followed in performing rescue breathing for adults:

Place hand under neck, thus lifting it and tilting the head back. Place one hand on the crown of the head tilting it backward so that the throat is stretched tight. Pull the chin up. This prevents obstruction of the tongue.

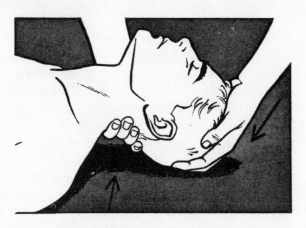

Take a *deep* breath. Open your mouth *wide*.
Mouth-to-Mouth Breathing

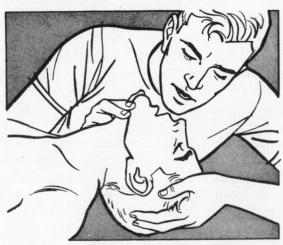

Place your mouth tightly over victim's mouth. Fold his lower lip down to keep his mouth open during inflation and exhalation. To prevent leakage, pinch his nostrils closed or press your cheek against his nostrils. Blow vigorously into the victim's mouth—hard enough to make his chest rise.

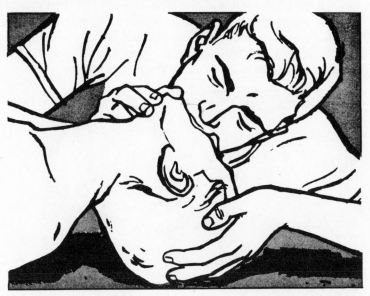

Mouth-to-Mouth   Mouth-to-Nose

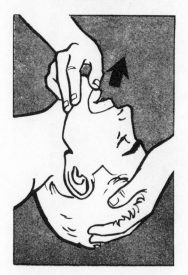

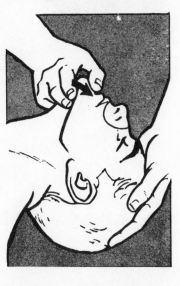

Remove your mouth. Listen for the sound of returning air. If you don't hear it, quickly sweep your fingers through his mouth to remove any obstruction, then tilt his head back farther and try to inflate his lungs again.

Breathe into his mouth again. If you still get no air exchange, turn victim on his side and slap him between the shoulders to dislodge foreign matter. Quickly return to breathing for the victim. Take your next breath as you listen to the sound of his breath escaping. Reinflate his lungs as soon as he has exhaled. Continue inflations at least twelve times each minute.

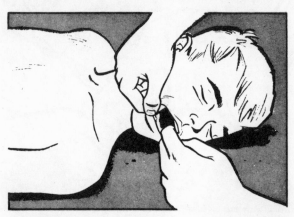

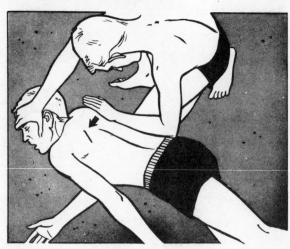

Mouth-to-Nose Breathing

Seal your lips widely on the victim's cheeks around the nose. Be sure your lips don't close his nostrils. Close his mouth with your thumb on his lower lip. (See illustration p. 155.)

If his head is not tilted enough, the soft palate allows inflation through the nose but exhalation through the mouth. If this happens tilt more, or part his lips with your thumb after each inflation.

The choice between mouth-to-mouth and mouth-to-nose breathing usually is not important. However, in some instances only one of these methods will work. Use mouth-to-nose breathing if victim is convulsing, if his mouth is difficult to open, or if his stomach gets inflated too much during mouth-to-mouth breathing. Use mouth-to-mouth breathing if the nasal passage is blocked, or if you have to use one hand to control the victim's body (in the water for instance).

RESCUE BREATHING FOR INFANTS AND CHILDREN

Properly administered, the new resuscitative techniques may be applied to the tiniest premature infant with spectacular success. Within minutes a blue, flaccid baby can be turned into a pink, wriggling newcomer.

Whenever possible place the infant on his back. You may use the back seat of a car, a table, or the floor. However, if necessary, you can do rescue breathing with the infant in your lap.

Lift the neck gently and tilt the head back until the skin over the throat is stretched. Place hand under neck. With the other hand, pull the chin upward, keeping the lips slightly open with your thumb. This is absolutely essential for keeping the air passage straight and open.

Open your mouth wide. For babies and very young children cover both nose and mouth tightly with your mouth. Take short puffs, about twenty a minute. It takes only a little air. Stop blowing as soon as the chest starts to rise.

Remove your mouth and let him breathe out by himself while you breathe in fresh air. It's time for the next breath as soon as you hear him breathe out. If there is no movement of the

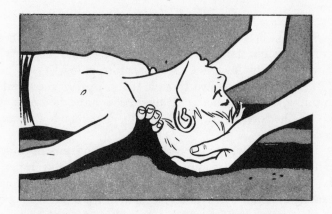

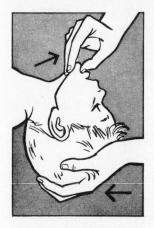
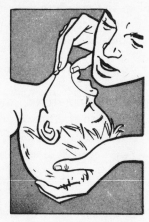

chest, hold him up by his ankles, open his mouth and let any
fluid or solids fall out or momentarily suspend the child head
down over your arm. Apply several sharp pats between the
shoulder blades. Then clear his throat with your fingers. Resume
rescue breathing immediately. As long as breathing is continued
a child can survive the presence of a coin, small toy, or food
particles in the throat until the obstruction can be removed in
the hospital.

In performing rescue breathing for an older child, you may
use either the nose or the mouth when you cannot cover both
with your mouth.

If excess air is blown into the stomach, some children will burp by themselves. In others, air is noted by an increasing bulge of the stomach between the ribs and naval. To remove air, press the victim's stomach gently. Check the throat for stomach contents before the inflation.

Prevent accumulation of excess air by keeping one hand on the stomach. Keep the head lower than the chest to prevent fluids from entering the lungs.

Don't give up. Don't stop until he starts breathing himself or until a doctor arrives.

RESCUE BREATHING FOR DROWNING VICTIMS

In handling a drowning victim it is important that resuscitation be started as soon as possible—a ten-second delay may make the difference between a life and death. Rescue breathing can and must be started in the water—as soon as you can reach the victim's mouth with your mouth and you are able to stand with your head out of the water. If you are an expert swimmer, you may be able to start rescue breathing while treading in deep water. Detailed procedures are as follows:

On reaching the victim, hook either your right arm through his right armpit or your left arm through his left armpit. With this lock grip, you can hold his head tilted way back with your other hand on the crown of his head. If you tilt enough, his mouth will open, making mouth-to-mouth breathing effective.

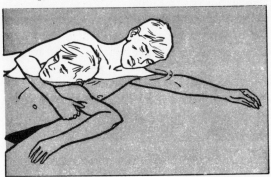

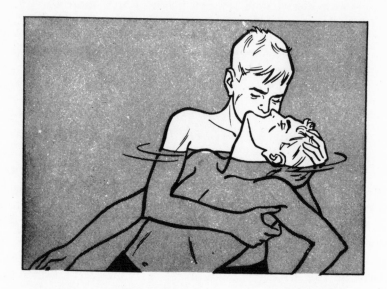

Because his body is lighter in the water, it's easy to lower him a little between breaths.

The first ten or twelve breaths should be given as fast as possible. Don't be concerned if the first few breaths cause water to spurt from his nose and mouth.

As you carry him ashore, breathe for him at least once every ten seconds. If he does not recover breathing by the time you reach shore, don't struggle to get him out of the water into the hot sun. The cool water reduces his need for oxygen, and in shallow water he's easier to pick up by stretcher or by hand when help comes. You can kneel in the water and rest his head on your knee. Now you can use both hands to hold his head tilted back fully and his chin pulled upward. In this position, you can switch from mouth-to-mouth to mouth-to-nose breathing if too much air is being blown into his stomach.

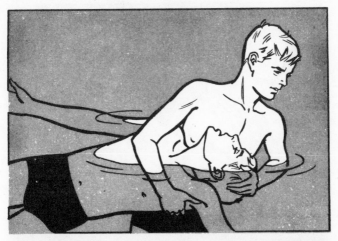

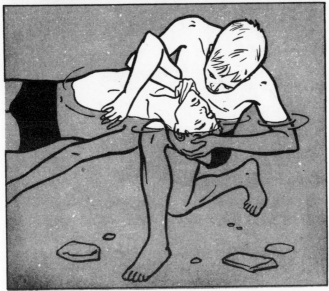

When he begins to recover, get him ashore so you can better care for him should complications arise. He may vomit food or sea water. If so, drain his throat each time to make sure the material does not enter his lungs. If possible, keep his head lower than his chest so any liquid will run out of his mouth.

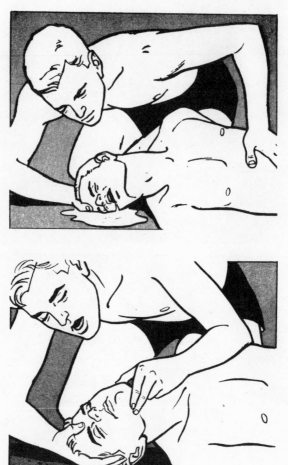

To aid this drainage, pull his shoulders over your knee to raise his chest. You may clean his throat of mucus or vomit or water with a cloth wrapped around your fingers.

During recovery the victim may have a convulsive seizure. If this happens, give him mouth-to-nose rescue breathing—enough to keep him pink. Watch his breathing carefully. If he lapses back to shallow breathing or turns blue, rescue breathe in rhythm with him. Continue rescue breathing until medical help takes over.

LEARN RESCUE BREATHING

Be prepared to breathe for your child, friend, and neighbor! Practice rescue breathing at home. Remember that you cannot hurt anyone by breathing for them. To avoid breathing against each other, get a third person to count 1 and 2 repeatedly. On the count of 1, the rescuer blows and the victim breathes in. On the count of 2, the rescuer takes in another breath while the victim breathes out. When the victim breathes with him, the rescuer learns what successful rescue breathing is. When the victim breathes against the rescuer or holds his breath, the rescuer learns what obstruction feels like. The victim should relax and let the rescuer do all the breathing for him.

Each member of the family should practice rescue breathing. It's too late to learn when the emergency arrives. Practice breathing with your child. First let him be the victim. Then let him "save" you.

Do not practice rescue breathing if you have a cold or infection. However, in an emergency, don't worry about infections. A life may be at stake. Start rescue breathing immediately. If you wish, you can cover the victim's nose and mouth with a piece of cloth, a handkerchief, the end of your shirt. The rescue breathing will still be effective. However, never use a cleansing tissue or a piece of paper to cover the nose or mouth while doing rescue breathing because they are nonporous and do not permit the air to get through to the victim.

YOUR OWN BREATH CAN SAVE A LIFE

Advantages of Rescue Breathing:
1. Rescue breathing works best in many situations because the victim does not need to be moved or placed on the ground.
2. Rescuer can get oxygen to victim's lungs faster than by any other known emergency method of artificial respiration.
3. Rescuer is in immediate contact with victim's face and breathing.

4. Both of the rescuer's hands are free to keep air passage open.
5. Rescuer sees, feels, and hears effect of each inflation.
6. Rescuer has big reserves of air and strength for inflating victim's lungs.
7. Rescuer can control the vigor of his effort to fit the size of his victim.
8. Small rescuer can breathe for large victim.
9. Rescuer can continue for hours without exhaustion.
10. No special equipment is needed.

EXTERNAL CARDIAC MASSAGE FOR ADULTS

If a pulse cannot be found by the rescuer external cardiac compression should begin immediately. If cardiac massage combined with rescue breathing is begun within three to five minutes after cardiac arrest, the central nervous system will receive enough oxygen to prevent serious damage. However, doctors warn that the quicker you are able to start resuscitation the better will be the chance of recovery.

The heart lies between the breastplate (sternum) and the spine. When pressure is applied to the sternum, the heart is compressed against the spine forcing blood into the arteries and pulmonary veins. Relaxation of pressure allows the heart to fill with blood. Because the thoracic cage in unconscious people is flexible the sternum can be depressed one and a half to two inches without endangering the ribs.

To determine the exact point to apply pressure, quickly locate the breastplate which lies in the center of the upper chest. The pressure point is on the lower half of the sternum above the soft lower end where it joins the abdomen. Place the heel of your left hand over the sternum—it should just fit since the bone is narrow. Throughout the entire procedure your lower hand is always in the same position—the heel of your left hand resting on the sternum. The heel of the right hand is placed over the left hand and pressure is applied by using your body weight. Pres-

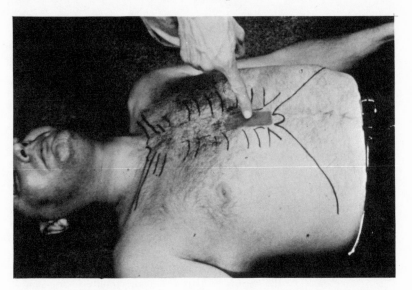

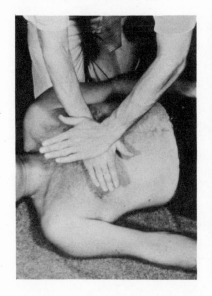

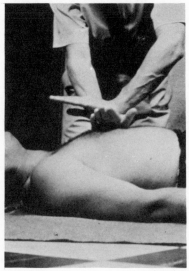

sure must be applied here and nowhere else if it is to be effective. Moving all over the chest or permitting the fingers—which should be kept raised—to come down can result in breakage of ribs and damage to internal organs. The procedure is as follows:

1. Place victim on his back on a solid surface—preferably the floor.
2. Kneel at the side of the victim so you can use weight of your body in applying pressure.
3. Place the heel of one hand on the lower half of the victim's sternum (breastbone) and the other hand directly on top of the other. Make sure that your fingers are opened and raised so that you will not depress the ribs which are easily broken.
4. With your arms in a vertical position, elbows straight, exert rhythmic pressure directly from your shoulder. Press down firmly at least an inch and a half to two inches. Make the downward stroke rapid, hold it for approximately one-half second.
5. Raise both hands after each manipulation to allow chest to expand.
6. Repeat this procedure once a second or somewhat faster (sixty to eighty times a minute).
7. Persist vigorously—patients have survived normally after three hours of external massage.

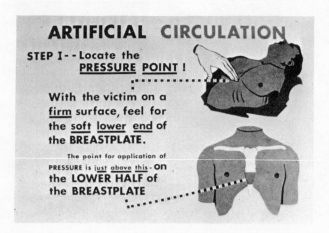

ARTIFICIAL CIRCULATION

STEP I - - Locate the PRESSURE POINT !

With the victim on a firm surface, feel for the soft lower end of the BREASTPLATE.

The point for application of PRESSURE is just above this - ON the LOWER HALF of the BREASTPLATE

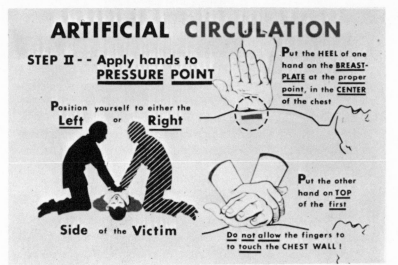

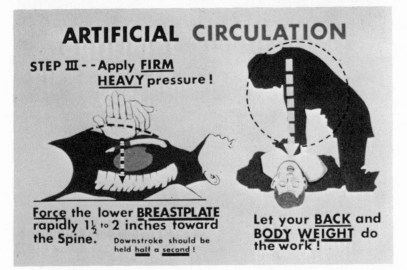

EXTERNAL CARDIAC MASSAGE FOR CHILDREN

1. Place an infant or very young child on a flat surface with his head toward you.
2. Use the tips of two fingers or both thumbs to gently compress the middle third of the sternum—a child's heart is higher than an adult's and the thoracic cage is more flexible.
3. If you use the thumbs, superimpose them over the middle of the breastbone. For additional support link the fingers behind the back of the baby.

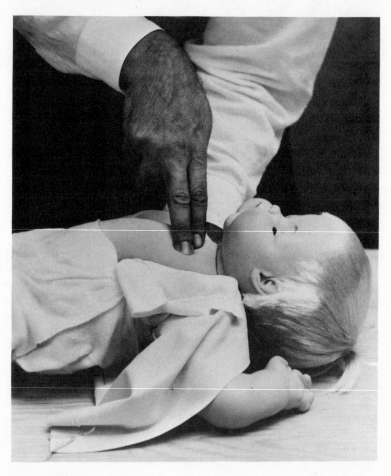

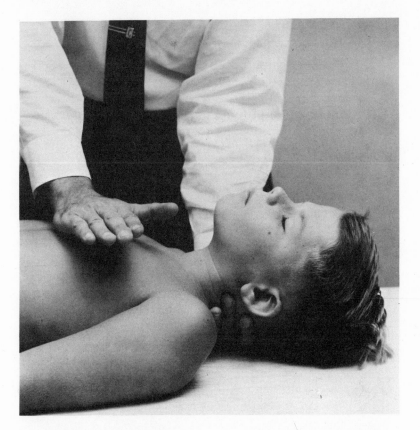

4. Compress the heart at the rate of 100 to 120 times a minute. If you're alone you can combine closed-heart massage with mouth-to-mouth breathing. Start by breathing several times for the baby using only puffs of air—hard blowing can injure the lungs. If the heart has definitely stopped, quickly start compressing the chest. It takes only a little pressure to compress the infant's heart. Pediatricians say that even if the heart has not entirely stopped closed-heart massage will do no harm.

5. If the child is under ten, use the heel of only one hand. Press down just hard enough to compress the chest the necessary two inches—the child's thoracic cage is still quite flexible. The rate of compression is between 100 and 120.

RESCUE BREATHING AND MANUAL HEART
COMPRESSION QUESTIONS AND ANSWERS

Q. How soon should mouth-to-mouth resuscitation be administered to a victim?

A. Immediately. The body tissues must receive oxygen within four minutes, otherwise damage will result to the tissues.

Q. When do you stop mouth-to-mouth resuscitation?

A. When the victim is breathing on his own.

Q. When is it *too late* to start direct breathing and external cardiac massage?

A. Unless you can be absolutely certain that more than six to ten minutes have passed since the victim's heart stopped beating, institute resuscitation procedures at once. Let a physician then decide whether resuscitation should go on or be stopped.

Q. Suppose we know that a drowning victim was in the water for at least fifteen or twenty minutes before being found. Should we try to resuscitate?

A. Yes. You don't know when the heart stopped beating. It may have stopped a quarter of an hour—or only seconds—before you found him.

Q. Suppose the victim is seventy-five years old, and is known to have been in bad health for some time. Should we try resuscitation?

A. Yes. Only a physician can determine that resuscitation should not be performed or continued because of the victim's state of health.

Q. What is the chance of contracting a contagious disease when applying mouth-to-mouth breathing?

A. None.

Q. How do you determine that the heart has stopped circulating the blood?

A. There are four signs:
>   1. Cessation of breathing
>   2. No pulse
>   3. Blue or very pale color
>   4. Dilation of eyes

Q. What does the blue color in a victim indicate?

A. Oxygen deficiency caused by cessation of breathing or stoppage of the heart.

Q. What if we can't feel any pulse, but the pupil contracts when we open the eye. Should we resuscitate?

A. Contraction of the pupil tells you that his blood is circulating and that his heart is beating. Therefore, you do not give him external cardiac message. But, if he isn't breathing, assist him with mouth-to-nose or mouth-to-mouth breathing.

Q. What if we feel a pulse, but the pupil doesn't contract?

A. If you can feel a strong pulse, the victim's heart is beating and he doesn't need external cardiac massage. But if he isn't breathing, assist him with mouth-to-nose or mouth-to-mouth breathing.

Q. Is it necessary to synchronize rescue breathing and manual heart compression?

A. Not necessary—mouth-to-mouth breathing should be performed twelve to sixteen times per minute; while manual heart compression is performed sixty to eighty times per minute.

Q. Is it necessary to first remove dental plates from the victim's mouth?

A. No. Start mouth-to-mouth breathing immediately. The dental plates should be removed only if they create a blockage or are loose in the mouth.

Q. Where there is only one operator, what is the sequence of applying mouth-to-mouth breathing and manual heart compression?

A. First apply five breaths, followed by fifteen compressions, then two breaths and fifteen compressions. Maintain that sequence of two breaths and five compressions until relieved. In other words, ventilate and circulate.

Q. Can this technique of rescue breathing and manual heart compression be applied to a pregnant woman?

A. Yes.

Q. Do we apply external cardiac massage and artificial respiration if the victim's chest has been badly injured or crushed?

A. Cardiac arrest resulting from crush injury to the chest is usually due to internal damage. External cardiac massage should *not* be performed.

Q. How long should resuscitation efforts be continued before we stop?

A. Resuscitation efforts should be kept up until a physician directs that they be stopped.

Q. Should we try to get a victim's heart going by giving him an electric shock, the way doctors do to defibrillate victims?

A. Absolutely not. Ordinary house current (115 volts), whether AC or DC, will actually put a heart into fibrillation rather than out of it. In fact, most cases of death due to electrocution are caused by this current. Defibrillation is a technique that requires special equipment, carefully selected voltages and amperages, and training that only physicians have had.

Q. Is it important to massage at the rate of exactly once a second?

A. No. Although once-a-second massage seems to be the optimal rate, massage that is performed a little faster or slower should be just about as effective.

Q. Which form of breathing is best? Mouth-to-nose or mouth-to-mouth?

A. You may use whichever you are trained in. If you use mouth-to-nose breathing, be sure that the victim's mouth is kept tightly shut; if you use mouth-to-mouth breathing be sure that his nostrils are held closed.

Q. Do we stop external cardiac massage and direct breathing while the victim is being driven to the hospital?

A. No. Resuscitation efforts should be continued every possible moment—on the ground, on the stretcher, in the ambulance, on the way into the hospital emergency room, and so on. No harm will be done by brief, unavoidable interruptions while the victim is being lifted or put down.

Q. What would you say we ought to watch out for most of all in external cardiac massage?

A. First—make sure that the victim actually needs it. If his heart is beating, he doesn't need external cardiac massage.
Second—be sure that you aren't breaking his ribs or damag-

ing his liver or other internal organs. Keep your fingers away from the victim's ribs, and apply the proper pressure in the proper place.

Third—external cardiac massage without mouth-to-nose or mouth-to-mouth breathing is useless.

Fourth—check frequently to find out whether the victim's heart and/or breathing have started again.

Fifth—don't get discouraged, and don't give up resuscitation unless a physician so instructs you.

"The number of lives we can save will be in direct proportion to the number of people who receive adequate training in modern resuscitation," states Dr. Leonard Scherlis, eminent cardiologist of Maryland University and member of the American Heart Association Committee on Resuscitation.

Today in many communities throughout America training in the new resuscitative techniques is being offered. Doctors train ambulance drivers, nurses, lifeguards, firemen, and police who often act as rescue squads. And some doctors have made independent efforts to teach closed-heart massage and mouth-to-mouth breathing to heart patients' families, who may find it difficult to get emergency help within three to five minutes.

But this is barely a start. Doctors maintain that what is needed is a program where every man, woman, or child would have a chance to learn the urgent techniques of modern resuscitation. The new life-saving skills require no medical background. "Anyone who is interested can learn to do them effectively," says Dr. Scherlis.

The crucial need for such training is made clear when we learn that the American Heart Association predicts that within the next five years one out of every seven men between the ages of forty-five and sixty-five will meet with sudden death. Experts believe that a trained American public would act as our first line of defense against sudden death, cutting these frightening statistics by 50 percent.

Experts point out that properly trained laymen acquit themselves with great skill and devotion in emergency situations. During World War II men and women were taught such sophisticated techniques as giving injections, stopping hemorrhages, and handling fractures.

In many hospitals resuscitation committees, usually headed by an anesthesiologist, give training courses. Though their first responsibility is to train hospital personnel, they often include lay people. Dr. Helene Mayer, associate clinical professor of anesthesiology at the New York University Medical School and attending anesthesiologist at Bellevue Hospital, New York City, has trained thousands of people to do cardiopulmonary resuscitation. In addition to training nurses, ambulance personnel, and other paramedical employees, she has taught classes of boy scouts, high school students, and clergymen.

A young nurse trained by Dr. Mayer recently stopped for gas. The owner of the station seeing her uniform begged her to help a man who had collapsed in the men's room. When the nurse bent over the stricken man who lay on the floor she could not detect any heartbeat nor was he breathing. She immediately started mouth-to-mouth breathing. Within a few minutes the man began to respond. His heart was beating and he was breathing on his own when the ambulance arrived.

The nurse told Dr. Mayer: "I used to think I would find it difficult to place my mouth over that of a stranger, but I found when the situation warranted it I did it without a qualm. It was wonderful to see the man responding."

How can you tell if a person is in clinical death or if he has just fainted? One sure way is to start resuscitation. If he has fainted, you will be unable to give either rescue breathing—he will fight you—or heart massage, which is far too painful if the patient is not completely unconscious.

Dr. Mayer believes resuscitation is definitely in order if the victim is obviously in distress—unconscious, face blue or deathly pale, breathing not apparent. Says Dr. Mayer: "It is true that some apparently dead patients may not be dead at all, that a mirror or a piece of cotton in front of the patient's mouth may show some slight movement of air, or that a stethoscope over the heart or an electrocardiogram may show some activity of the heart muscle. In that case the rescuer may get some undeserved credit. He may only have *kept* this person alive, not restored life; heart and lung activity was probably inadequate to maintain life."

In many cities the local branches of the American Heart Association provide training. The Los Angeles County Heart Association, which now holds or assists in some 250 sessions a year, is opening its classes to broader groups. Dentists, gym teachers, auto and truck drivers, elementary school teachers, and utility workers, selected because they are responsible for first-aid emergencies, have received training.

Because of the excellent work done by the Michigan Heart Association in training people, this area is one of the few in the United States where effective resuscitation techniques are usually applied when emergencies arise. The association has given instruction in resuscitation to twenty thousand physicians and nurses, police and firemen, water safety and industrial safety men. They are now extending their service to include any layman who wishes to learn.

One of the most comprehensive training programs was given recently in Pittsburgh, Pennsylvania, by Drs. Sidney W. Winchell and Peter Safar of the Department of Anesthesiology of the University School of Medicine. The trainees included young medical students, dental students, student nurses, college and high school students, and a church group of men and women. Teaching aids consisted of films, slides, booklets, graphs, and life-size mannequins. Lectures by the instructors were given with simultaneous demonstration of techniques. This was followed by supervised practice on a Resusci-Anne mannequin that simulates airway obstruction and flexion of the neck, chest movement with inflations, and a carotid pulse when the heart is compressed.

Feeling of the carotid pulse was demonstrated slowly and in detail on a semirecumbent volunteer and then on the mannequin.

All members of the class were asked to attempt palpation of the pulse in each other. Feeling of the carotid pulse was combined with maintenance of head tilt. Mouth-to-mouth and mouth-to-nose ventilation was demonstrated with emphasis on maximal backward tilt of the head, tight oral seal, and forceful blowing. The necessity to accompany external cardiac compression with active lung inflations was stressed. The entire sequence was demonstrated repeatedly.

For practice sessions the trainees were divided into groups of ten to fifteen volunteers per instructor. The instructors, resident anesthesiologists, supervised practice until each trainee performed the entire sequence of A, B, C (Airway opened, Breathing restored, Circulation restored) correctly without coaching. At the end of the teaching session trainees were told they would be called back for a "refresher session" and that their performance would be evaluated at that time. If necessary, they would be retrained.

When the trainees were recalled a month later, the instructors found that *the lay group who had diligently practiced performed better than the nonpracticed paramedical groups.* This proved the original theory of the physicians that it takes constant practice if the rescuer hopes to perform well in an emergency. It also made clear that resuscitation techniques can be readily learned by lay people.

During the period of evaluation the instructors found the most common causes of failure to ventilate were inadequate head tilt, inadequate oral seal, and inadequate force of blowing—in this order of frequency. The most common error in failure to circulate was "fumbling" (indecision), namely not producing an adequate number of compressions within the two minutes allotted for the test. Failure to diagnose pulselessness followed by use of potentially injurious hand position occurred in about 10 percent of all trainees tested. All trainees who passed the over-all mechanics test performed the first inflation within the first twenty seconds, the first sternal compression within ten to fifteen seconds later. Those who failed any part of the test took longer.

Dr. Safar and Dr. Winchell found that laymen who have had good training are capable of instructing classes as effectively as physicians. Training aids—films and film strips, diagrams, pictures, and most important of all a Resusci-Anne mannequin—can be borrowed from the local Heart group, the Public Health Service, or the Red Cross.

12.

THE LEGAL COMPLICATIONS

The legal complications that can ensue over the question "When is a patient dead?" were dramatized when a wealthy southern shipowner recently met with a catastrophic accident. Rushed to a hospital, it was found that he was clinically dead on arrival. A team of doctors immediately took over and expended heroic efforts to resuscitate him. They succeeded in getting the heart to beat weakly and kept it going erratically for forty minutes. But at that time the doctors recognized that complete resuscitation was impossible and he was pronounced dead.

Meanwhile, during the same critical forty minutes, a baby girl was born to the shipowner's only daughter. The daughter had married against her father's wishes. As a result, he had disowned her, but had set aside $100,000 for any grandchild who might be born before his death.

Was the new baby entitled to the inheritance? Was her grandfather dead when he got to the hospital or was he alive?

By traditional standards he was dead, for the law recognizes death when the heart stops and respiration ceases. But the doctors were able to make his heart beat during the forty minutes when the baby was born. The law specifically says that a heartbeat connotes life. Therefore, was he really dead when he was brought into the hospital?

This case was settled out of court. But such questions will arise again until there is a new ruling on what constitutes death.

Though the law is slow to change—many of our current laws involving death go back to the seventeenth century—the verdicts brought in by juries and the briefing by judges make it clear that they are basing their decisions on current practices. Physicians who have not promptly used resuscitative techniques to revive patients on operating tables are apt to find they are guilty of criminal negligence.

More than 3,500 years ago the Code of Hammurabi suggested that a doctor who opened a man's body and caused his death or treated his eye and caused loss of sight should have his hand cut off. Since those harsh days, the meaning of malpractice has changed considerably. Generally speaking, it now means faulty or bad practice on the part of a doctor that leads to injury and is clearly below the standard of practice in the area in which he is practicing. To prove that a doctor has acted unskillfully, however, opposing medical testimony is needed—that is to say, one doctor must testify that another has deviated from accepted medical standards.

But because of the difficulty of getting one doctor to testify against another, a new legal development is becoming accepted practice in our courts. Known by its Latin name, *res ipso loquitor,* "the thing speaks for itself," this concept is making acceptable the results of gross medical error as proof of malpractice.

It is estimated that nationwide at least one out of six doctors is being sued or has been sued. In some parts of the country—California, Minnesota, the District of Columbia, Alaska, and Oregon (areas of hyperactivity in malpractice suits)—the figures may be closer to one out of four. Experts estimate that this year costs, fees, court-awarded damages, and settlements may approach $75 million.

Because of the severe damage that can occur when sudden death is not dealt with promptly and expertly, juries are inclined to have great sympathy for the victim. Legal cases growing out of cardiac arrest have brought some of the biggest jury awards and settlements recorded in years.

"The public is aware of the fact that you needn't die when

your heart stops," points out Howard Hassard, who serves as counsel for the California Medical Association as well as its executive director. "Now they expect doctors to be able to perform resuscitation without any bad results."

There was a bad result when an Oakland opthalmologist undertook surgery on a six-year-old-boy to correct an inward deviation of the eyes. Suddenly the surgeon heard the anesthesiologist call out: "His heart has stopped." The anesthesiologist quickly let the anesthetic mixture out of the reservoir bag, refilled it with oxygen and began closed-chest massage. The ophthalmologist watched anxiously as the other physician pressed the boy's chest and relaxed, pressed and relaxed.

After about a minute, when the child failed to respond, the anesthesiologist asked the surgeon to open the chest and massage the heart manually since this often works when the closed-chest massage doesn't.

"I can't," the ophthalmologist replied. "I'm not qualified for the procedure—I've never done it before." Instead of trying, he rushed out and grabbed a passing surgeon.

The second surgeon opened the boy's chest and got the heart beating again. But too much time had passed. The boy is now blind, mute, and a quadruple paraplegic.

The parents, maintaining that they had sent to the hospital a boy and got back a vegetable, brought suit. The malpractice trial that followed hinged on these questions: Was the patient a good surgical risk? Did the defendant physicians handle the emergency according to the prevailing standard of care in the community? If so, was the prevailing standard itself a negligent one?

Expert medical witnesses for the defense testified that the prevailing standard of care in the community did not require an ophthalmologist to be competent to perform open-chest massage. The plaintiff could produce no medical witness to dispute them. Still, all the doctors who took the stand agreed that cardiac arrest was a known risk of surgery, and an operating doctor should be prepared to deal with it in some way.

In briefing the jury the Court pointed out that some time prior to this incident the county medical society had presented lectures, movies, and demonstrations on the problem of cardiac arrest and how it should be handled. The information that open-chest massage should be used if closed-chest massage proves ineffective was included. These courses were open not only to members of the society but also to specialist groups, such as ophthalmologists. Plaques explaining the techniques were put up in all the operating rooms.

The Court told the jury that it could infer that proper standards required a surgeon to have some knowledge of how to perform resuscitation. If he has not had proper training, then he must have someone standing by who can immediately take over in case of heart arrest.

The Court concluded, "The thing speaks for itself. There was negligence."

The jury found against the surgeon and the hospital for $400,000. An appeals court reversed the verdict. It said the case should never have gone to the jury, since no expert witness testified that the doctors had been negligent. But the California Supreme Court ordered a new trial. Even without expert testimony for the plaintiff, the Supreme Court said, there was enough evidence for the jury to assume negligence. Rather than take their chances with another jury, the surgeon and the hospital settled the case out of court for $255,000.

California's Supreme Court isn't the first court to react sternly to a surgeon's failure to correct cardiac arrest. In Florida a surgeon was performing an abdominal operation on a thirty-two-year-old woman, the wife of a Navy chief petty officer, when her heart suddenly stopped.

The surgeon ordered an intravenous feeding of norepinephrine—a drug used to stimulate the beat of the heart. There was no reaction. Then he injected the drug directly into her heart chamber. Still no response. Finally after considerable time had passed, he got another surgeon to open her chest and massage her heart. But it was too late to prevent brain damage.

The patient was left in a condition similar to that of a permanent paraplegic. Her condition is pathetic. For a year and a half she was fed by tube. Later, she was able to eat only pureed foods. She can stand upright, if assisted, but cannot walk. She cannot talk, except for an occasional word. She is sensitive to pain and can indicate where she hurts. She can understand questions, which she answers by moving her head or winking signals for yes or no. This doctors believe is the extent of improvement possible.

In a judgment of $78,500 to the damaged patient a U.S. District Court said: "A surgeon undertaking a surgical procedure should possess as part of his qualifications the ability to perform a thoractomy (opening of chest) and manual cardiac massage."

In awarding the settlement, the court estimated that the cost of future medical care would be $115 a week and that she had a life expectancy of ten years. Apart from the injury, her life expectancy would have been forty years. The compensation granted for future medical expenses was $48,500. Other elements of compensation were $4,000 for past pain and suffering; $15,000 for future disability; and $10,000 to the husband for his past and future loss of the companionship and services of the patient.

Dr. Valentino D. B. Mazzia, chief of anesthesiology at Bellevue Hospital Center in New York City, says that in many types of cardiac arrest the closed-chest technique doesn't work while the open-chest method does. A surgical team unprepared to perform a thoractomy, he warns, is confronting a known risk of surgery without being prepared with the most effective weapon to combat it. Help from the operating room next door, he points out, is often "too little and too late." And tardiness in a case of cardiac arrest, the courts are saying, may equal negligence.

Dr. Robert H. Smith, who heads the Department of Anesthesiology at the University of California Medical School, recently reported that many patients are dying unnecessarily because their doctors do not know how to restore their breathing or keep their airways open.

Dr. Smith gave the case history of an eighteen-year-old football player who died while having a broken nose set by two general practitioners. The doctors used tetracine-soaked wedges in the smashed bony ledges within the nose to provide local anesthesia. There was nothing complicated about the break and since the boy was a husky specimen whose health had always been excellent, there seemed little reason for apprehension.

But the anesthetic was so rapidly absorbed that it produced vascular collapse that quickly progressed to cardiac arrest. The football player who had come in with a broken nose was clinically dead. Neither of the physicians knew how to use modern methods of resuscitation to restore breathing. In desperation they called the fire department. But by the time the firemen arrived the boy was beyond recall.

Courts and medical authorities have also delved in the surgeon's responsibilities before and after surgery. In one case a surgeon ordered an anesthetic for a patient about to undergo a mastoidectomy, then left the operating room. The patient's heart stopped, but the anesthesiologist managed to get it going again with epinephrine. Under the circumstances the surgeon decided not to go ahead with the operation. Later, the patient was found to have suffered brain damage.

In the suit that followed, the surgeon claimed he couldn't be held negligent, not having been present when the accident occurred. Actually a surgeon is always supposed to be present when anesthesia is administered.

However, since no expert witness had testified that it was standard practice for the surgeon to be in attendance when anesthesia was being administered, the defense moved for dismissal. The Court refused the motion.

"It is no hardship on the physician," said the judge, "to explain how the injury occurred and why he was not present to prevent it."

Under certain conditions the surgeon's legal responsibility extends into the recovery room. In New York, a surgeon completed a routine tonsillectomy without incident and escorted the patient, a twelve-year-old boy to the recovery room. With the patient apparently in good condition, the surgeon left.

Minutes later, the boy stopped breathing. A nurse—the only professional person in the room—called the surgeon and the anesthesiologist. They rushed back to the recovery room with a thoracic surgeon in tow. The chest man cut into the boy's pleural cavity and started his heart. But it was too late to prevent extensive brain damage. The parents sued for $1,500,000. Eventually, the surgeon, the anesthesiologist, and the hospital settled the case out of court for $300,000.

Sometimes it's the anesthesiologist rather than the surgeon who is the target for a criminal negligence suit. In a California case, a general practitioner administered the anesthesia while the surgeon performed an abdominal operation on a thirty-seven-year-old woman for removal of a ruptured and gangrenous appendix. While the last sutures were being put in to close the incision, the absence of pulse or blood pressure was noticed by the anesthesiologist, who turned off the flow of nitrous oxide, commenced a flow of pure oxygen, and squeezed the bag to help the unconscious patient to breathe.

The surgeon had an assistant perform closed-chest massage and then performed a thoractomy. The anesthesiologist did not perform an intubation—putting a tube of oxygen into the trachea.

The heart resumed its normal beat and the incision was closed. The patient's brain, however, had been without sufficient oxygen for from four to six minutes. Brain damage resulted.

The woman was left almost completely incapacitated. Bedridden, she can answer yes or no to questions by blinking her eyes. She can show contentment when her husband or children visit her by making a cooing sound. She can indicate displeasure by crying. Otherwise, she is incapable of any human activity.

During the trial that followed, a specialist in anesthesiology testified that the use of an indotracheal tube is virtually mandatory at a time when a thoractomy is being performed. Another general practitioner who frequently administers anesthetics stated his opinion that any physician who as a substantial part of his practice acts as an anesthesiologist must be competent to handle an intubation under the prevailing standard of medical practice. There was also expert testimony that cardiac arrest occurs in abdominal surgery in about one case in ten thousand but that the incidence is much lower with the best of care.

The physician charged with negligence in this case admitted that this was the proper standard of medical practice. He also admitted he was not qualified to intubate a patient.

Nevertheless, the jury exonerated the general practitioner-anesthesiologist, but the decision was reversed on appeal. The reviewing court held that the testimony was sufficient to require an instruction that would permit the jury to infer negligence in the absence of evidence that would satisfactorily explain how the injury occurred without negligence.

The general practitioner in this case faces a new trial unless a further appeal is taken or a settlement is made.

Richard P. Bergen, a member of the law department of the American Medical Association, points out that these decisions illustrate two important facts of life in the legal aspects of medical practice: First, the risks of an adverse decision are very high when medical treatment has a tragic and unexpected outcome. Second, every medical practitioner must, at his peril, be professionally competent and adequately prepared to cope with the complications that are known to occur in the procedures he undertakes.

One result of the spate of malpractice suits is that some doctors are becoming so defensive that they are reluctant to handle certain cases. In Rhode Island, a husband and wife—both doctors—were brought to court for refusing to get involved in an emergency. In Brooklyn, an internist refused to help a man wounded by gunfire and was suspended for a month by his medical association. Other doctors simply prefer to drive without MD plates on their cars.

Actually their excuse, that if they stop to offer aid to an injured person they might eventually find themselves involved in a lawsuit, doesn't hold water. The Good Samaritan law, which in twenty-six states is rated as excellent and is adequate in the rest of the country, protects the physician who offers help to a stranger. A member of the American Medical Association legal department points out that as far as they knew no one had ever been successfully sued in this country when they volunteered help to a person in trouble. He bluntly adds: "It is often used as an excuse by doctors."

Actually it is the patient who is in jeopardy, according to attorney George E. Hall, a staff associate in the AMA law department. Writing on the value of the Good Samaritan laws, he recently stated: "These statutes grant physicians special privilege of nonliability for their careless acts, and grant no substitute right to the injured party—not even the right to demand the emergency medical care for which the doctor is granted negligence immunity." Attorney Hall suggests an alternative legislative possibility. "Lawmakers might want to consider a statute that would require a physician to stop and render aid in return for exemption from some liability."

David Cleary, science writer on the Philadelphia *Bulletin*, recently gave an eyewitness account in which fifty-seven-year-old Robert Boomer, of Muncie, Indiana, lay on the sidewalk in front of the Park-Sheraton Hotel in New York for forty-five minutes awaiting the arrival of a police car and an ambulance.

Mr. Cleary, while keeping vigil with Mr. Boomer, was able to identify six passersby as doctors who were attending the forty-seventh annual meeting of the American College of Physicians two blocks away. Not one of the doctors stopped to offer help. When Cleary asked one of the men whose badge was sticking out from under his raincoat to help the prostrate man, he reacted by pulling his raincoat completely over the badge, thus hiding his name. He told Cleary: "I'm not licensed in New York State" and hurried into the Park-Sheraton Hotel through an entrance a few feet away.

Fortunately it turned out that Boomer was not in grave medical danger. At the city-operated Roosevelt Hospital, where he arrived fifty-three minutes later, doctors could find no evidence of a heart attack or other serious ailment. Their only finding was that he had cracked three ribs when he fell. They taped his chest so the ribs would heal and released him.

New York has an excellent Good Samaritan law that protects doctors against lawsuits whenever they provide first aid or emergency treatment away from hospitals and their offices, as long as they act in good faith and are not grossly negligent. New York's law applies to "any duly-licensed physician or surgeon."

Mr. Cleary makes the point that few convention-going doctors are well versed in the laws of the state in which their conventions are held. Rather they are motivated—or not motivated—by their medical training, personal emotions, and what they would customarily do.

13.

CRYONICS—THE ULTIMATE IN RESUSCITATION

The resuscitation techniques that are practiced today throughout the civilized world are merely a foreshadowing of what the future will bring. As a result of basic research now in progress, scientists plan to use hypothermia—the freezing of cells and tissue—to preserve the lives of men, not for decades but for centuries. People who have died of incurable diseases will be immediately frozen into "suspended death" until such time as medical science learns to correct their pathological abnormalities. They will be thawed, their ailments cured, and they will then be returned to life.

This far-out planning is not forecast for a hundred years from now. It is already with us. In many countries, including the United States and the Soviet Union, it is possible right now to place a person who has entered clinical death into suspended animation. In the United States six men and four women have already been frozen and their bodies placed in freezer capsules to be preserved at the coldest possible level until such time as they can be restored and returned to the world.

Scientists predict that within a decade freezing people who die of incurable ailments will become standard procedure and that all hospitals will one day be equipped with freezers where bodies can be kept until they can be given a second chance at life.

The promise of hypothermia is especially meaningful to

parents who face the heartbreaking experience of losing a child to death from an incurable disease—a disease that in all probability may be conquered within the next few years. With hypothermia there could be the solace and hope that by putting the child into suspended death it would eventually be cured and have a chance to live the life that was cut short.

The chief drawback at present with placing a person in a frozen state for an extended period is the uncertainty of effective thawing. When freezing is continued for a long period, there is apt to be damage to the central nervous system. Scientists are now working to find the means to return a person from suspended death without any injury or with damage so minimal that it can easily be corrected.

In the Soviet Union, where research on hypothermia is a major project, they are experimenting with, and hope soon to have available, a medical mixture that will delay all vital processes and the disintegration of the vital organs and tissues without interfering too deeply with the functions of the central nervous system. Such a medical development would make suspended death an accepted medical routine as well as providing great prospects for medicine and surgery in general.

Scientists who have recently visited the Soviet Union are of the belief that it is already using hypothermia to preserve their more important comrades who die of diseases that are presently incurable. The new Russian hospitals are equipped with pump oxygenators, hypothermia machines, and pressure chambers—resuscitation implements that would be helpful both in the freezing and eventual thawing. The staff is trained to use this equipment and is available at all hours to put it in operation if the need arises.

The beneficial effects of cold have been known to man for centuries. Primitive man used applications of cold to reduce the heat of fever and to alleviate swelling and infection. In the early 1600s Marcus Aurelius Severinus, noted surgeon of his day, often applied globs of snow and ice to extremities before amputating. This type of anesthesia was revived when Napoleon's armies suffered a crushing defeat as a result of Russia's severe cold. Baron J. D. Larrey, his chief surgeon, observed that half-frozen soldiers survived amputations and other trauma much better than comrades protected from the cold.

To achieve the bridge from our present life span and the future-projected longevity, scientists will use cryobiology—low temperature biology. The study of the physics of extreme low temperature scale in this relatively new branch of science involves a degree of cold that might be found on the dark side of the moon. It ranges all the way from —150° Fahrenheit down to absolute zero or —489° Fahrenheit. This is the coldest possible cold—the point at which all molecular motion ceases.

In this frigid domain fantastic things happen. Air turns to liquid or freezes as solid as a block of ice. Steel becomes as brittle as glass and electrical resistance drops to zero. A rubber ball shatters on impact. Most of life's processes come to a halt, without the finality of death.

Experiments in the use of hypothermia to prolong the short span of clinical death were begun ten years ago in the laboratories of Experimental Physiology for Resuscitation of the Soviet Academy of Science. Scientists discovered that when hypothermia was used, the energy potential of the brain after thirty minutes of cardiac arrest is equal to that of five or six minutes at normal temperature. Animals whose blood had been completely drained and were in clinical death could be revived with all their functions intact after an hour if they were kept cooled at 77° Fahrenheit.

Further experiments established the fact that as the temperature was lowered, the cells of the brain and other tissues became more resistant to the effects of death. When placed in hypothermia at 50° F., the vital functions of animals—dogs and monkeys were used—could be completely restored after two hours. Testing nerve cells, which are particularly vulnerable to the process of death, they found that the lower the temperature the longer the period of clinical death could be prolonged.

Monkeys proved more sensitive to the cessation of circulation than dogs. The vital functions were restored only in some monkeys while all the dogs were revived. However, monkeys who did recover did so much more quickly. After thirty minutes of clinical death under hypothermia, it took two or three days for a dog to completely come back, while monkeys were alert within six or eight hours after revival.

Kafa, an eight-year-old female baboon, was the subject of one of the early experiments. She was clinically dead; there was no heartbeat or respiration and all of the blood had been completely drained from her body. At the end of half an hour, resuscitation was started. Blood was pumped back into Kafa's veins and artificial respiration was undertaken. After fifteen minutes, Kafa began breathing on her own. Four hours later, she opened her eyes and lifted her head. When doctors tried to give her penicillin injections, she seized the syringe and began running around the operating room. Her outward appearance and general behavior differed little from that of a healthy animal.

Later, when they gave Kafa some tangerines, she chose the sweet ones and threw away the sour ones, and when offered candy, she chose the varieties that had been favorites before the experiment. Scientists concluded that a monkey's brain, when protected by hypothermia, seems able to compensate for and resist the process of dying. The monkey's reactions, researchers find, more closely resemble those of man than those of any other animal. When a human being is resuscitated, the cortex usually becomes active within one to twenty minutes after the heart starts beating.

Dr. Negovsky, the famous Soviet scientist who sparked much of the present-day research in hypothermia, recently reported the case history of a farmer who was resuscitated after three hours of clinical death. Vladimir Kharin, a tractor driver on a farm in Tselinny territory, was caught in a snowstorm and his tractor stopped. For two hours, while the temperature continued to fall and the snow grew heavier, he tried to repair the tractor. But finally, his hands numb and his strength all but gone, he had to give up.

Kharin started back on foot to the state farm which was ten kilometers away. He kept falling into snowdrifts, half blinded with the snow, his body frozen. As he collapsed for the last time, completely exhausted, his last thought before losing consciousness was that he was only twenty-three, that he had a wife and a small daughter, and he wanted to live.

Several hours later, a crew of workmen from the Yaraslavsky State Farm in Aktyubinsk Region found the body of Kharin lying in a snowdrift. He seemed dead. His frozen fists were tightly clenched and his stiff body sounded hollow and wooden against the floor of the truck that took him to the hospital. Doctors found that both heart and respiration had stopped, that the pupils of his eyes did not react to light. They were interested, however, in the fact that his skin, instead of being the usual corpselike pallor, was a bluish-purple color, and there were no signs of putrefaction. Theorizing that he might still be in a state of clinical death, they decided to attempt to save him.

Kharin's feet were placed in warm water to dilate the vessels, his arms and body were rubbed with alcohol, and adrenalin was injected into the heart muscle to stimulate heart activity. Blood was pumped into his arteries, followed by artificial respiration when the tissues became softer. After forty minutes, signs of life could be detected. His skin became warm and his pulse began to beat feebly. More blood was pumped into the artery and Kharin was laid in a sterile bed and warmed with hot water bags. Consciousness returned twelve hours later. He was able to tell doctors that he had lain for three hours in the snow. After several months in the hospital, Kharin recovered sufficiently to return to his job.

Dr. Negovsky makes the point that this case does not seem incredible as it is a well-known fact that life can be restored after several hours of clinical death if the body temperature is reduced to 50°-53.6° F. under special conditions, particularly under narcosis. Kharin was in a state of deep hypothermia. When he lost consciousness, his breathing became slow and superficial and carbon dioxide tended to accumulate in his blood. This is the very narcotic that has been used in experiments to cause artificial hibernation in warm-blooded animals.

The field of research in human freezing is young and moving fast. It offers high drama and controversy, holds out hope as well as serious problems that are gradually being solved. But even while researchers continue to seek ways in which hypothermia can be used with safety for extended periods, it has already proved its value on many life-saving fronts.

Hypothermia is bringing surgery to a new level of expertise; it is curing ailments that formerly responded only to surgery if at all; and it is restoring to normality people who have suffered brain damage during prolonged clinical death or through injury.

Today cryosurgery—deep freezing of tissue (its name comes from the Greek word *kryos*, meaning ice cold)—is replacing the scalpel in operating theaters throughout the country. Instead of cutting, the surgeon simply freezes tissue and bone ice-hard with a device called a cryoprobe—a hollow tube in which liquid nitrogen circulates at a far below-zero temperature. The frozen cells die and are subsequently removed either by the surgeon or, more commonly, by the body's own waste-disposal system.

With the use of cryosurgery, operations that once took hours can now be completed in minutes; the patient requires only local anesthesia; the possibility of operative and post-operative hemorrhage in some types of surgery is all but eliminated. Often the patient can walk out of the hospital within hours. But the most amazing thing about cryosurgery is its versatility.

The technique of cryosurgery was pioneered in 1961 by Dr. Irving Cooper, director of neurosurgery at St. Barnabas Hospital, New York, to relieve the rigidity and uncontrollable tremors of Parkinson's disease by freezing a tiny cluster of nerve cells inside the brain. The patient is given a local anesthetic and a dime-size hole is cut into his skull. Guided by a series of Polaroid X rays, Cooper inserts a probe the size of a crochet needle into the thalamus, about two and one half inches deep in the brain.

A ball of frozen tissue gradually forms around the tip and, since the patient is conscious, Cooper can gauge the effect by observing his hand movements. The procedure is safe, because if the ice ball grows too large and the patient shows signs of paralysis, the doctor has thirty seconds to raise the probe temperature and avert permanent damage.

Cryosurgery is being tested increasingly in other types of surgery. Dr. Cooper, for example, has frozen brain tumors that are too deep in the brain to be removed by conventional methods. After destruction by freezing the dead tumor breaks down and is removed by the bloodstream.

At the Buffalo, New York, VA Hospital, Dr. Andrew Gage has frozen bone tumors by wrapping a freezing coil around the bone shaft. The dead bone forms a structure around which new bone forms, Dr. Gage reports. Dr. Maurice J. Gonder, also of Buffalo VA, and his associate Dr. Ward A. Soanes have found the cryosurgical probe a good way to remove the prostate gland with relatively little pain and blood loss. And Dr. William G. Cahan of New York's Memorial Hospital has used cryosurgery to remove tonsils, to stop abnormal uterine bleeding (by destroying the lining of the uterus), and to relieve pain from large incurable tumors. The technique is also used in head and neck surgery, and to freeze semen for later use in artificial insemination.

The most exciting aspect of cryosurgery has been its effective use in treating many types of cancer. At the State University of New York School of Medicine in Buffalo, this type of surgery has been used successfully on more than sixty patients with cancer of the skin, tongue, mouth, throat, bone, or rectum. The malignancies in some cases had resisted X-ray treatment.

Many could not have been removed surgically without extensive loss of bone.

It was during the treatment of prostate cancer that one of the most important values of cryosurgery was discovered. In some patients the cancer was far advanced and had begun to spread beyond the prostate. But after freezing the prostate tissues, physicians discovered that not only was the cancer destroyed but shrinkage of cancerous tissues in other areas had taken place. Studies now under way suggest that freezing somehow causes the body to produce antibodies—defense agents—against cancerous tissue, and these antibodies, traveling via the bloodstream, may attack cancerous tissue wherever it exists.

It also acts as a powerful deterrent to the spreading of cancer cells. For example, a tumorous mass about to be excised is frozen to fix the malignant cells in position and prevent their inadvertent release into the surrounding tissue and circulatory avenues where malignancies could arise.

Dr. Cahan makes the point that the first clinical trials of cryosurgery were undertaken out of desperation. The hospital had many patients hopelessly sick with cancer that had proved resistant to surgery, irradiation, chemotherapy, cauterization, or combinations of these methods.

In a series of 120 cases, which included several types of carcinoma in many areas of the body, cryosurgery was used. A number of the conditions yielded gratifying results.

Dr. Morris Fishbein, writing in *Medical World News* about the use of cryosurgery, states:

> In the brief period during which this new technique has been studied in many hospitals and clinics, the enthusiasm usually associated with the new methods has grown steadily. Time will be required for more accurate evaluation, but certainly what has already been accomplished offers hope for the treatment of many cases that would be considered virtually incurable with older methods.

Techniques in the use of hypothermia are constantly improving. Only two or three years ago it was considered remarkable to freeze a person for twenty or thirty minutes in order to perform a difficult operation. Doctors now routinely freeze debilitated patients who face critical surgery for two or three hours, thereby assuring full protection to the vital organs.

Dr. Alfred Uihlein, of the famous Mayo Clinic in Rochester, Minnesota, recently reported on a series of operations where patients were put into deep freeze while repairs were made on intracranial aneurisms—an outpouching or ballooning in the wall of an artery that usually results in death. Dr. Uihlein said that by cooling the body to a temperature less than 64.4° F., a bloodless field was established and maintained for as long as an hour. Yet "despite the magnitude of the procedure, comparison of the degree of neurological deficit before and after operation indicated that the use of hypothermia and circulatory arrest produced gratifying results."

But it is hypothermia's great potential for lengthening the life span that makes it a prime subject for researchers. Dr. Bernard L. Strehler recently announced that if human temperature could be reduced just three degrees, the average man might live twenty years longer. Dr. Strehler, director of the biological laboratory at USC's Rossmoor-Cortese Institute for the Study of Retirement and Aging, said it has been established that cold-blooded animals age more slowly at reduced body temperatures.

We do not know whether this rule applies to warm-blooded animals such as ourselves. If it does, however, the effect of reducing our body temperature from 98.6° Fahrenheit to 95.6—a small change well within the range of fluctuations we have all experienced—would be to add about twenty years to the average life expectancy.

The use of hypothermia to extend life not for hours, days, or weeks, but for centuries, becomes more important in view of the many medical discoveries that are being developed. For there is no doubt that within this century many of the great killers of mankind will have been made obsolete by new knowledge and fresh techniques of medical science. By arranging to have themselves frozen into "suspended animation," the bold experimenters are buying a unique form of insurance to prolong their life.

Nor are these pioneers of a new movement martyrs to science. Their present potential life span will remain unaltered by even a day or an hour. And they leave this world with the solace that they may return again to the only universe they know.

Although the whole conception of freezing a patient while he's in clinical death and returning him to life years later is still radically new, it has caught the imagination of people all over the world. Cryonics societies have sprung up in many parts of the United States and Europe. Many of their members have already made provision to have themselves and their loved ones quick-frozen and stored in cryocapsules as a gamble on future rescue from death. They believe that before long such non-funerals will become commonplace.

The first person to have himself quick-frozen in this country was Professor James H. Bedford, a psychology professor who died January 12, 1967. Professor Bedford, who was seventy-three, was firm in the belief that by having himself frozen he was participating in an experiment that would have tremendous value to humanity. So great was his faith that he left a $100,000 for the endowment of the Bedford Foundation, which will do cryogenic research. He also left money to build a mausoleum in California for the storage of those frozen with the hope that virtual immortality awaits them. Both his wife and son had agreed to the experiment.

At the dying man's bedside, was a four-man medical team of the California Cryonic Society. In the hospital room ready to be put to use as soon as death took over was a heart-lung machine, profusion equipment—to interchange blood with chemical solutions—an iron heart (a heart and lung resuscitator), and a variety of drugs that would be used to freeze the body.

As Professor Bedford lapsed into a coma, Dr. B. Renault

Able, who headed the medical team, began packing ice around him in an effort to reduce his body temperature. Twenty minutes later the heartbeat and respiration failed. Professor Bedford was clinically dead. Dr. Able, assisted by Dr. Robert Prehoda, director of research for the Bedford Foundation, Dr. Dante Brunnol, of the University of Southern California, and Robert Nelson, president of the Cryonic Society of California, immediately began the eight-and-one-half-hour freezing process. While Dr. Able started external heart massage to keep the brain alive other members set up the heart-lung machine and readied other equipment.

To prevent clotting, heparin, an anticoagulant, was injected into the body. When the professor's body temperature dropped to 46.4° F., most of the blood was removed from his body and a mixture of 85 percent Ringer's solution and 15 percent DMSO (dimethyl sulfoxide) was substituted. When the profusion was finished, the body was suspended in dry icy vapors, which gradually lowered its temperature to −174.2° F.

Then the body, in a state that cryobiologists call "suspended death," was transferred into a temporary styrofoam-insulated box packed with dry ice. A death certificate listing lung cancer as the cause of death was signed and arrangements made to ship the body to Phoenix, Arizona, where a cryocapsule—a cryonic suspension unit—had been ordered from the Cryo-Care Equipment Company, one of several firms that manufacture freezer capsules for the storage of bodies for an indefinite length of time.

A week after the professor's death, his body, wrapped in aluminum foil, and the stretcher upon which it rested was inserted into the inner cylinder of the cryocapsule which had been cut open for the purpose. The strange coffin, resembling a giant thermos bottle, was then hermetically sealed and liquid nitrogen poured through a valve that lowered Bedford's body temperature to an incredible 428° below zero—so cold that in the unlikely event the body should be dropped, it would shatter like glass.

The cryocapsule is so heavily insulated that its shiny white outer surface remains at room temperature despite the extreme cold inside.

The liquid nitrogen that is poured in evaporates very slowly through an escape valve, which also prevents pressure build-ups that might otherwise cause an explosion. A series of gauges along the capsule's surface keep track of the amount of coolant and warn of any significant temperature change. Since no electricity is involved, power failures are no danger to the experiment. Nitrogen is added to the capsule every four to six months, depending on how rapidly it evaporates.

Bedford's capsule will be returned to California for long-term storage. The cost of the freezing and the perpetual care runs to about $10,000. Members of cryonics societies are urged to take out insurance policies that will provide for the necessary expenses involved in keeping a body in deep freeze until it can be cured of its ailments and restored to life.

Eventually it is hoped that multiple storage of patients will be used, thus cutting down the cost of the process. In fact, one member of the New York Cryonics Society, which has several hundred members, is working on a huge cryogenic container that could hold twenty to forty bodies.

How long will the body of Professor Bedford remain in the capsule? Two scientific developments must take place before he can be resuscitated. A complete cure for cancer of the lung, which was the cause of his death, must be found. And researchers working in laboratories must come up with a safe method of thawing a human being who has been deeply frozen.

According to doctors and cryobiologists, who study the effect of extreme cold on living organisms, the professor's body could remain frozen in its hermetically sealed capsule indefinitely, up to hundreds of years if necessary. But cryobiologists say the chances are excellent that within a decade there will be a cancer cure and the knowledge of how to freeze and then thaw a body will be available.

The youngest and the most poignant of those who have been frozen until he can safely be returned to life is twenty-four-year-old Steven Mandell, who died in New York City on July 28, 1968. Steven was a student at New York University where he majored in aeronautical engineering.

Ever since Steven was eleven years old science in all its phases had been an overwhelming interest. "He began by building every spaceship model he could lay his hands on," his mother, Mrs. Pauline Mandell, recalls. His parents encouraged him because he added to the kits, made innovations that were his own invention.

A creative and imaginative boy, "he read voraciously on scientific subjects and planned a career in that field."

Steven was only eighteen when he first became ill. He was stricken with enteritis, a painful disease which usually strikes in middle or later life, especially among those who experience intense inner stress. But the irony of Steven getting the disease was that he was a happy, outgoing adolescent with an active, meaningful life.

In 1966, when Steven's health was much improved and it looked as if he might be able to lead the life of a normal, healthy boy, he saw an advertisement for the Cryonics Society in a science-fiction magazine. It featured the slogan of the society: "Never Say Die!"

Science-oriented Steven was immediately interested. He showed the ad to his girl friend. "I want to be in the vanguard when science fiction turns into science fact," he told her.

He sent for an application blank. With it he enclosed the following note: "Although financially limited at the moment I am fully committed to the Cryonics movement and will contribute all that I can to its progress and acceptance." He reported his health as being fair.

His recurring illness and subsequent death came suddenly. His doctor found the sudden collapse unexplainable, fought desperately for Steve's life. Everything that science knows about the disease was brought to bear. But to no avail. The doctor told Mrs. Mandell that her son was dying.

Even as a terrible numbness seemed to seep through her

body, she remembered that Steven had told her that if he died he wanted to be frozen—that he hoped it would give him another chance at life which he loved so well. She had reassured him and promised him that of course she would remember. But she had not believed for a moment that there would be any need; Steven had undergone other sieges that had been far worse than this. Faced with the brutal fact of his impending death she needed to act. Her son had left a telephone number with her. Now she phoned the Cryonics Society of New York, told them that Steven was dying, that his last wish was that he be frozen at death.

Steven died early Sunday morning. From the first minute members of the society took over, made all the arrangements. His clinically dead body was quickly moved to the mortuary of Columbia Presbyterian Hospital where it was kept under refrigeration. A mortician in St. James, Long Island, was immediately contacted. He came in with an air-conditioned hearse. Steven was packed in cubes and bags of dry ice for the two-hour journey to the Long Island mortuary. There his body was further chilled and perfused—a freezing liquid was inserted in his veins and arteries to prevent the formation of ice crystals. Resuscitation to keep his brain alive was continued throughout the hours that he was being prepared for internment.

Having made all the arrangements for Steven, Mrs. Mandell was faced with another problem. Steven obviously could not have a "funeral" in the ordinary sense because he was only clinically dead. But though neither she nor Steven were very religious, her husband, who had died when Steven was seventeen, belonged to an Orthodox Jewish congregation. She felt that if it were at all possible there should be a religious ceremony for Steven. The problem was how to find a rabbi who would agree to it. Steven was dead in the medical sense, within the over-all limitations of present knowledge. But in this time of organ transplants and open-heart surgery, even clinical death has become a clouded area. Would any rabbi agree to officiate at memorial services for her son under these conditions?

It was the members of the Cryonics Society that found an understanding rabbi, Bernard A. Rubeinstein. He told the bereaved mother, "I can't see anything wrong with cryonization from the religious point of view. Religion deals with our souls; if we have a soul it enters paradise when it leaves the body after death. I see nothing sacrilegious in cryonic suspension at all. I believe religion and science must work much more closely together."

Forty-five relatives and friends gathered to say good-bye to Steven, who at this time was in a temporary container filled with dry ice at a temperature of −110° Fahrenheit. On Thursday, September 5, 1968, Steven was transferred to a cryocapsule, a permanent unit where he will remain until such time as it is felt that he can safely be returned to the world he loved. Stored with him are his complete medical records and a tape recording he made shortly before he died in which he recorded his interests, beliefs, and philosophic development. His unit is being maintained at Washington Memorial Park in Coram, Long Island.

Mrs. Mandell says: "I don't want people to think that I *know* my son, Steven, is going to come back to life. I let the Cryonics Society freeze his body, rather than having it interred or cremated, because it was what he wanted. When his father died he said to me at the cemetery, 'Ma, if I go first, don't put me under the dirt. Eventually there's nothing but the earth itself.'

"If there's one chance in a million that he will come back—or even if *my son* doesn't have it—if he can help somebody else to have it—what have we lost?

"Even if it occurs sometime in the future, that I may not live to see the day—it is easier for me to bear his untimely death because there wasn't the same finality as that of putting him away underground."

Hypothermia as a measure to extend life is no more radical

than an iron lung, the use of miracle drugs, or the transplanting of the human heart, say cryobiologists, and they point out that all of these recent medical developments have been fully accepted. But whether it is possible to thaw a person who has been deeply frozen and bring him back to life is a question that has triggered bitter debate in the scientific world.

Robert C. Ettinger, formerly a physics professor at Highland Park Community College in Detroit, Michigan, and adviser to the medical team who froze Professor Bedford, rates the chances as excellent.

"There is good reason to believe that most of the cells of his body are still alive, and this is the basis of the project," declares Ettinger, who has already made elaborate plans to have himself, his wife, and their two children quick-frozen upon their death.

But other medical authorities, among them Dr. John Lyman, head of the biotechnology laboratory at UCLA, and Dr. Stanley Jacobs, associate professor of surgery at the University of Oregon Medical School, disagree vehemently.

Said Lyman, accusing the experimenters of failing "to think the problem through": Freezing has a cataclysmic effect on the fine structure of cells, disrupting their chemical and physical nature and making it extremely doubtful that life can be restored. He adds:

"The process of thawing prevents simultaneous thawing of all organs, resulting in deterioration of the more rapidly thawing body parts, while others warm at a slower rate. There's a lot of research on this general subject but we just don't have the technology, especially with larger animals or humans."

Said Jacobs, who took an even bleaker view of the whole idea: "It is not possible by present methods to do what they are attempting to do. Once he's frozen, he's dead and he's not going to come back again."

But criticism doesn't seem to dismay advocates of the freezing theory. They point to British work with half-frozen golden hamsters, who recovered normal activity, and Japanese experiments on the brain of a cat that was frozen at −4° for 203 days. When thawed, it registered a normal encephalogram reading.

Cryobiologists and physicists such as Ettinger and Able tend to regard death as a purely temporary condition, one that future scientists will be able to control, even though present ones cannot.

Their argument is that we can avoid death now through freezing and wait, patiently entombed, for the day when science will know how to bring us back from the grave. Taking the chance, they say, is better than dying outright.

Ettinger says: "Storage in liquid nitrogen will keep the body essentially unchanged for an indefinite period, except for some minor freezing damage. If our optimism proves justified, and we do learn how to cure or repair all damage—including the physical disability of old age—then people who die now will have indefinitely extended life in the future."

Dr. Able points out that if we can assume that it is possible to freeze a piece of tissue—and it is—then we can safely assume it could be done with a whole animal.

And Professor Jean Rostand makes the flat statement that "most of us now breathing have a good chance of physical life after death—a sober, scientific probability of revival and rejuvenation of our frozen bodies."

Many scientists agree with Professor Rostand that the freezing of people during clinical death must be regarded as an excellent gamble, with little to lose and an enormous prize to gain. There is general optimism that as freezing methods are improved the chances become more favorable.

E. Wesley Walten, of Converse College, has said: "The time draws near when men will be unchained from the birth-death cycle. We owe it to our own concept of courage to try. It is a good thing and an heroic thing, and a rare and farsighted human thing to join in what one might call hand-to-hand combat with death itself."

Resuscitation and hypothermia are part of the surging, newly awakened spirit of this scientifically oriented century. Scientists urge that the important thing with which we must concern ourselves is what we want from the future—not what the future will be doing for us. For the future cannot be predicted, but it can be invented.

Author's note:

The word "cryonics" was suggested four years ago by Karl Werner, vice president of the Cryonics Society of New York. Although etymologically rooted in the Greek *kryos* (cold) along with "cryogenics," it is the latter term that has taken on, somewhat inappropriately, the meaning of low-temperature science and technology. "Cryonics," on the other hand, refers specifically to the process of suspended animation by the use of hypothermia. While the disciplines and programs centered on human cold storage are known by relatively few scientists, the term "cryonics" is enjoying an ever-widening acceptance.

INDEX